VOLUME ONE HUNDRED AND THIRTY ONE

ADVANCES IN
CANCER RESEARCH

KV-036-925

VOLUME ONE HUNDRED AND THIRTY ONE

ADVANCES IN
CANCER RESEARCH

Edited by

KENNETH D. TEW

*Department of Cell and Molecular Pharmacology,
Medical University of South Carolina, Charleston,
South Carolina, United States*

PAUL B. FISHER

*Department of Human and Molecular Genetics,
VCU Institute of Molecular Medicine, and VCU Massey
Cancer Center, Virginia Commonwealth University,
School of Medicine, Richmond, Virginia, United States*

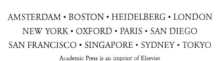

AMSTERDAM • BOSTON • HEIDELBERG • LONDON
NEW YORK • OXFORD • PARIS • SAN DIEGO
SAN FRANCISCO • SINGAPORE • SYDNEY • TOKYO
Academic Press is an imprint of Elsevier

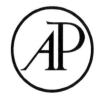

Academic Press is an imprint of Elsevier
50 Hampshire Street, 5th Floor, Cambridge, MA 02139, United States
525 B Street, Suite 1800, San Diego, CA 92101-4495, United States
The Boulevard, Langford Lane, Kidlington, Oxford OX5 1GB, United Kingdom
125 London Wall, London, EC2Y 5AS, United Kingdom

First edition 2016

ISBN: 978-0-12-804788-0
ISSN: 0065-230X

For information on all Academic Press publications
visit our website at https://www.elsevier.com/

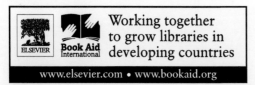

Working together
to grow libraries in
developing countries

www.elsevier.com • www.bookaid.org

Publisher: Zoe Kruze
Acquisition Editor: Zoe Kruze
Editorial Project Manager: Sarah Lay
Production Project Manager: Surya Narayanan Jayachandran
Cover Designer: Matthew Limbert

CONTENTS

4. AEG-1/MTDH/LYRIC: A Promiscuous Protein Partner Critical in Cancer, Obesity, and CNS Diseases   97

L. Emdad, S.K. Das, B. Hu, T. Kegelman, D.-c. Kang, S.-G. Lee, D. Sarkar, and P.B. Fisher

5. Role of the RB-Interacting Proteins in Stem Cell Biology   133

M. Mushtaq, H. Viñas Gaza, and E.V. Kashuba

6. Evolving Strategies for Therapeutically Targeting Cancer Stem Cells   159

S. Talukdar, L. Emdad, S.K. Das, D. Sarkar, and P.B. Fisher

CONTRIBUTORS

S.K. Das
VCU Institute of Molecular Medicine; VCU Massey Cancer Center, Virginia
Commonwealth University, School of Medicine, Richmond, VA, United States

G. David
NYU Cancer Institute, New York University School of Medicine, New York, NY,
United States

D. Dupéré-Richer
Division of Hematology Oncology, The University of Florida Health Cancer Center,
Gainesville, FL, United States

L. Emdad
VCU Institute of Molecular Medicine; VCU Massey Cancer Center, Virginia
Commonwealth University, School of Medicine, Richmond, VA, United States

T. Ezponda
Division of Hematology/Oncology, Centro de Investigacion Medica Aplicada (CIMA),
IDISNA, Pamplona, Spain

P.B. Fisher
VCU Institute of Molecular Medicine; VCU Massey Cancer Center, Virginia
Commonwealth University, School of Medicine, Richmond, VA, United States

C.A. French
Brigham and Women's Hospital, Harvard Medical School, Boston, MA, United States

C. Hajdu
New York University School of Medicine, New York, NY, United States

B. Hu
Virginia Commonwealth University, School of Medicine, Richmond, VA, United States

D.-c. Kang
Ilsong Institute of Life Science, Hallym University, Anyang, Republic of Korea

E.V. Kashuba
Karolinska Institutet, Stockholm, Sweden; R.E. Kavetsky Institute of Experimental
Pathology, Oncology and Radiobiology, NASU, Kyiv, Ukraine

T. Kegelman
Virginia Commonwealth University, School of Medicine, Richmond, VA, United States

S.-G. Lee
Cancer Preventive Material Development Research Center, Institute of Korean Medicine,
College of Korean Medicine, Kyung Hee University, Seoul, Republic of Korea

J.D. Licht
Division of Hematology Oncology, The University of Florida Health Cancer Center, Gainesville, FL, United States

W.H. Miller Jr.
Segal Cancer Centre and Lady Davis Institute, Jewish General Hospital, Division of Experimental Medicine, McGill University, Montreal, QC, Canada

M. Mushtaq
Karolinska Institutet, Stockholm, Sweden

J.N. Nichol
Segal Cancer Centre and Lady Davis Institute, Jewish General Hospital, Division of Experimental Medicine, McGill University, Montreal, QC, Canada

A. Porciuncula
NYU Cancer Institute, New York University School of Medicine, New York, NY, United States

D. Sarkar
VCU Institute of Molecular Medicine; VCU Massey Cancer Center, Virginia Commonwealth University, School of Medicine, Richmond, VA, United States

S. Talukdar
Virginia Commonwealth University, School of Medicine, Richmond, VA, United States

H. Viñas Gaza
Karolinska Institutet, Stockholm, Sweden

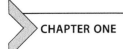

CHAPTER ONE

The Dual Role of Senescence in Pancreatic Ductal Adenocarcinoma

A. Porciuncula*, C. Hajdu[†], G. David*,[1]

*NYU Cancer Institute, New York University School of Medicine, New York, NY, United States
[†]New York University School of Medicine, New York, NY, United States
[1]Corresponding author: e-mail address: gregory.david@nyumc.org

Contents

Abstract

The role of senescence as a tumor suppressor is well established; however, recent evidence has revealed novel paracrine functions for senescent cells in relation to their microenvironment, most notably protumorigenic roles in certain contexts. Senescent cells are capable of altering the inflammatory microenvironment through the senescence-associated secretory phenotype, which could have important consequences for tumorigenesis. The role of senescent cells in a highly inflammatory cancer like pancreatic cancer is still largely undefined, apart from the fact that senescence abrogation increases tumorigenesis in vivo. This review will summarize our current knowledge of the phenomenon of cellular senescence in pancreatic ductal adenocarcinoma, its overlapping link with inflammation, and some urgent unanswered questions in the field.

1. INTRODUCTION

1.1 Pancreatic Ductal Adenocarcinoma: An Overview

Pancreatic cancer has one of the most dismal survival rates of all cancers due to its late presentation and resistance to current therapies (Ryan, Hong, & Bardeesy, 2014). While other cancers can now be detected early and/or adequately treated, if not stably eradicated, pancreatic cancer has always been incomprehensibly difficult to manage in the clinic and remains incurable. In the United States, incidence almost equals mortality, and its incidence rate is steadily on the rise with 53,070 new cases and 41,780 deaths expected to occur in 2016 (Siegel, Miller, & Jemal, 2016). Its peculiar biology, anatomical location, and the lack of treatment options tailored to the disease may explain its failures in the clinic. All this warrants a deeper understanding of its pathogenesis and biology.

The most common type of pancreatic cancer is pancreatic ductal adenocarcinoma (PDAC), which arises in the exocrine compartment of the pancreas. Histologically, PDACs are characterized by ductal differentiation, hypovascularity, and strong desmoplasia (Neesse, Algul, Tuveson, & Gress, 2015). They are usually accompanied by numerous ductal lesions termed pancreatic intraepithelial neoplasias (PanINs), believed to be the precursors to the cancer (Hruban, Goggins, Parsons, & Kern, 2000). According to the progression model, normal ductal epithelium develops into PDAC passing through PanINs 1 to 3, with increasing degrees of cytoarchitectural and nuclear atypia (Table 1), with PanIN-3s generally considered as ductal carcinoma in situ (Hruban et al., 2004). Genetic studies seem to support such a model as higher grade PanINs harbor similar mutations to those found in PDAC: namely in the four genes *KRAS*, *p16/CDKN2A*, *TP53*, and *DPC4/SMAD4* (Feldmann, Beaty, Hruban, & Maitra, 2007).

Technical developments in genetic engineering allowed the generation of mouse models that faithfully recapitulate human PDAC while supporting the PDAC progression model. The analysis of these models of PDAC has led to significant advances allowing the study of physiological processes during disease evolution and the means to assess potential preclinical therapeutic

Table 1 Guide to Classification of Lesions in the Pancreas

	Normal Duct	ADM	PanIN-1	PanIN-2	PanIN-3	PDAC
Histology	Cuboidal to low columnar	Tubular (bulging lumen); ductal parenchyma	Columnar; flat (PanIN-1A) or papillary with focal slight pseudo stratification (PanIN-1B)	Mostly papillary; prominent nuclear stratification of the full thickness of epithelium	Papillary; budding off into lumen; luminal necrosis	Invasive; stromal reaction
Visible mucin	–	–	+	+	–	–
Nuclei	Normal	Normal	Basally located, round, smooth contour	Enlarged, crowding, hyperchromatic, Smooth contour Small nucleoli; mitosis rare, basally located, morphologically normal	Enlarged, hyperchromatic, irregular contour; prominent nucleoli; mitosis usual, including atypical forms	Enlarged, hyperchromatic, irregular; prominent nucleoli; mitoses
Atypia	–	–	–	+/++	+++	+++
Loss of polarity	–	–	–	+/focal	+++ complete	+++
Mutations						
KRAS	–[a]	+[b]	+	+	+	+ (>90–95%)
P16	–	–	±	+	+	+ (>90–95%)
TP53	–	–	–	–	+	+ (>50–75%)
SMAD4	–	–	–	–	+	+ (50–55%)
Senescence	–	+[c]	+[d]	–	–	–

[a]*KRAS* mutations, however, have been detected in rare normal duct cells of patients without pancreatic disease (Lutges et al., 1999).

[b]*KRAS* mutations have been observed only in ADMs associated with PanINs, not in isolated ADMs (Shi et al., 2009).

[c](Caldwell et al., 2012; Guerra et al., 2007).

[d](Caldwell et al., 2012; Carrière et al., 2011; Collado et al., 2005; Guerra et al., 2011; Rielland et al., 2014).

interventions (Pérez-Mancera, Guerra, Barbacid, & Tuveson, 2012). Expression of oncogenic Kras ($Kras^{G12D}$) driven by its endogenous promoter in pancreatic epithelia during embryogenesis using pancreas-specific Cre driver mice leads to formation of PanIN-like lesions and, in a small proportion of mice, invasive and metastatic adenocarcinomas that resemble human PDAC in terms of histology and markers (Hingorani et al., 2003). When coupled with inactivation of tumor suppressors commonly mutated in human PDAC, most notably Trp53, $p16^{INK4A}/p19^{ARF}$, and Smad4, tumors acquire a more invasive phenotype establishing higher penetrance of metastatic PDAC and significantly shortening median survival in these mice (Aguirre et al., 2003; Hingorani et al., 2005; Ijichi et al., 2006). These mouse models are promising tools for studying early and metastatic stages of PDAC pathogenesis.

1.2 The Biological Relevance of Cellular Senescence

Cellular senescence represents one of the early and primary defense mechanisms of a cell when faced with a stressor, such as an oncogenic mutation. A senescent cell undergoes a stable loss of proliferative capacity despite stimulation by proproliferation signals (eg, mitogenic or oncogenic stimuli), and maintains a metabolically active state (Kuilman, Michaloglou, Mooi, & Peeper, 2010). The origins of the stressors that can trigger senescence are diverse: serial passaging, oxidative stresses, oncogene activation, tumor suppressor loss, exposure to chemotherapeutic agents, tissue repair, aging, and certain developmental processes (Muñoz-Espín & Serrano, 2014). There is no one definitive marker of senescence. Its multifarious hallmarks include: senescence-associated beta-galactosidase (SA-β-gal) positivity, $p16^{INK4A}$ upregulation, activation of a DNA damage response, formation of senescence-associated heterochromatic foci (SAHFs), and the production of a senescence-associated secretory phenotype (SASP) (Sharpless & Sherr, 2015) (Table 2).

In the context of cancer, oncogene activation causes senescent cells to withdraw from the cell cycle, thus preventing their uncontrolled proliferation in a process called oncogene-induced senescence. Consistently, senescent cells have been identified in preneoplastic lesions, and, conversely, have been shown to be absent in full-blown cancers. More importantly, inactivation of senescence effector programs (eg, p53 and $p16^{INK4A}$ pathways) leads to increased tumorigenesis in vivo, indicating that senescence represents an important barrier to the malignant progression of tumors (Collado &

Table 2 Commonly Used Senescence Markers

Marker	Description	Utility In Vivo?	Used in Human PDAC Tissue?
SA-β-gal	Lysosomal stress detected at subacidic pH (Dimri et al., 1995; Kurz, Decary, Hong, & Erusalimsky, 2000)	+	−
p16 upregulation	Cell cycle inhibitor (Serrano, Hannon, & Beach, 1993)	+[a]	+
Activated DDR	Checkpoint response to correct DNA lesions (Di Micco et al., 2006), detected as DNA damage markers/foci or SAHFs (Narita et al., 2003)	−	−
SASP	Secretion of proinflammatory cytokines, growth factors, matrix-remodeling enzymes (Coppé et al., 2008)	+	−

[a]Current antibodies are poor in detecting p16 by IHC in mice (Sharpless & Sherr, 2015).

Serrano, 2010). However, what happens to senescent cells during cancer progression remains largely unknown. Studies on mouse models have shown that senescent cells, through their ability to secrete the SASP, can be cleared by specific populations of immune cells (Iannello, Thompson, Ardolino, Lowe, & Raulet, 2013; Kang et al., 2011; Xue et al., 2007), whereas a minority of them are believed to bypass or escape senescence contributing at least in part to tumor formation either by acquiring more mutations or by yet unidentified mechanisms (Kuilman et al., 2010).

While generally believed to be a protective mechanism of the cell against cancer, senescence has recently been shown to serve a paradoxically pro-tumorigenic function, which has been attributed to the SASP (Coppé, Desprez, Krtolica, & Campisi, 2010). The SASP converts senescent cells into proinflammatory cells which, depending on the microenvironmental context, could have favorable or deleterious effects on tumorigenesis. Accumulating evidence indicate that the SASP may also have protumorigenic effects, including the stimulation of cancer cell proliferation, motility, and the generation of an inflammatory environment that promotes tumor growth. In an inflammation-driven cancer like PDAC, the SASP may reveal unique features of the cancer resulting from the interactions of senescent cells with a highly inflammatory microenvironment.

This review will focus on an apparently dual role that senescence plays in pancreatic cancer: first, as a barrier against tumorigenesis (in a mainly cell-autonomous manner), and, also, as a proinflammatory process that modulates the tumor microenvironment (via its paracrine function), whose complex effects on tumorigenesis will be discussed.

2. SENESCENT CELLS IN PANCREATIC CANCER

2.1 Senescence in Pancreatic Tumor Cells

Senescent cells in the pancreas have first been detected within early grade PanIN lesions of 6- to 8-month-old pancreata of mice that express oncogenic Kras from its endogenous promoter (Collado et al., 2005). Within these lesions, some cells stain positive for senescence markers p16, Dec1, and DcR2; conversely, normal ducts and PDAC are negative for these markers (Collado et al., 2005). About 10% of cells comprising PanIN-1 are senescent based on expression of the standard senescence marker SA-β-gal; by contrast, senescent cells are rarely detected in corresponding PanIN-1 cells of p53-deleted PDAC mice, pointing to a requirement for p53 in Kras-induced senescence (Caldwell et al., 2012). These SA-β-gal-positive cells are negative for proliferation marker Ki67 (Caldwell et al., 2012; Carrière et al., 2011; Guerra et al., 2011; Rielland et al., 2014), and exhibit concomitant upregulation of senescence effector p16^{INK4A} and p53/p21^{CIP1} (Eser et al., 2013). At the same time, a similarly abundant population (>10%) of SA-β-gal-negative and Ki67-positive cells also exists within PanIN-1 lesions (Caldwell et al., 2012), suggesting the coexistence of senescent and proliferative cells within early grade PanINs in these mice. Of all the senescence markers described elsewhere, SA-β-gal appears to be the most robust for pancreatic neoplasias in mice (Caldwell et al., 2012).

Few studies have reported senescent cells in human PDAC, most of which corroborate findings obtained from mouse models (Caldwell et al., 2012; Guerra et al., 2011). According to these studies, human PanINs also stain positive for some of the senescence markers, such as p16^{INK4A} (Guerra et al., 2011), but have not been shown to be significantly enriched for these markers relative to human PDAC (Caldwell et al., 2012). This discrepancy could be explained by the fact that most human PDAC samples are far too advanced in progression that senescence most probably could have subsided in these tissues, even within the PanIN lesions found in the vicinity of the PDAC. Human PanINs, regardless of histological grade, have also been shown to uniformly (96% of PanINs analyzed) contain shorter telomeres, one of the earliest genetic alterations that occur in preneoplastic PDAC and that are conserved in invasive adenocarcinoma (van Heek et al., 2002). However, the potential causative link between telomere shortening and senescence in human PanINs remains to be formally determined. Overall, these findings point to potential differences between mouse and human PDAC progression at the level of senescence markers, and the need to validate mouse observations in human tissues (McDonald, Maitra, & Hruban, 2012).

2.2 Senescence as Barrier to PDAC Progression

As in other cancers, senescence has been shown to be an important barrier to cancer progression in PDAC. Genetic inactivation of key senescence effector pathways cooperates with oncogenic Kras to accelerate tumorigenesis and promote a metastatic PDAC, underlining the tumor suppressor function of senescence. Preliminary reports have focused on *Cdkn2a* and *Trp53*, also the two most commonly mutated genes in PDAC with *Kras*. Genetic inactivation of the *Ink4a/Arf* locus in oncogenic Kras-expressing pancreata accelerates PanIN formation, PDAC progression and promotes metastasis (Aguirre et al., 2003). Similarly, a dominant-negative $Trp53^{R172H}$ mutation introduced into the endogenous mutant Kras background promotes a metastatic PDAC with 100% penetrance, marked by gross chromosomal instability (Hingorani et al., 2005; Morton, Timpson, et al., 2010). These data suggest that key senescence effectors may not only restrict PDAC progression, but under certain circumstances (eg, $Trp53^{R172H}$ mutation) may also promote metastasis, a possibility that remains to be investigated. Taken together, these pathways constrain PDAC progression (Bardeesy et al., 2006) and prevent the progression of oncogenic Kras-expressing PanINs into frank PDAC.

2.3 Senescence Bypass in PDAC

Senescence bypass has been described as a mechanism by which preneoplastic PanIN cells are able to reenter the cell cycle and further contribute to PDAC formation. Of note, while senescence was first believed to be irreversible, acute somatic inactivation of retinoblastoma (Rb), a key senescence effector, in senescent fibroblasts has been shown to be sufficient to promote reentry in the cell cycle and proliferation (Sage, Miller, Perez-Mancera, Wysocki, & Jacks, 2003). In PDAC, Rb deletion accelerates tumorigenesis (Carrière et al., 2011). Surprisingly, PanIN cells in these pancreata undergo a stage where they simultaneously exhibit positivity for senescence markers (SA-β-gal, p16) and the proliferation marker Ki67, suggesting that Rb-deleted PanINs can initiate the senescence program, but cannot undergo growth arrest, and thus bypass the senescent state.

Activation of the AKT pathway, a downstream target of oncogenic Kras, suppresses Kras-induced senescence in the pancreas leading to a more aggressive PDAC (Kennedy et al., 2011). Interestingly, administration of mTOR inhibitor, rapamycin, restores senescence in these lesions; however, the therapeutic implications of such findings have not yet been explored. Lkb1 haploinsufficiency, a common mutation in PDAC, also exacerbates cancer progression in the mouse, correlating with the suppression of p21-mediated growth arrest (Morton, Jamieson, et al., 2010). All these observations underline the need for oncogenic Kras to cooperate with downstream mutations, whose main outcome appears to allow the bypass of the senescent state.

Certain physiological stimuli, like pancreatitis, also appear to promote tumorigenesis in PDAC by means of a senescence bypass (Guerra et al., 2011). The loss of senescence markers characterizes lesions of pancreatitis-driven PDAC in mice wherein oncogenic Kras is either activated during embryogenesis or adulthood. Notably, withdrawal of the pancreatitis-causing agent, caerulein, even for just a month, restores senescence in these lesions. Importantly, this finding, along with the rapamycin-restored senescence (Kennedy et al., 2011), suggests that senescence bypass could be reversible; however, in these models, it is not clear whether senescence is induced de novo or by reversion in previously senescent cells. Finally, senescence bypass has also been reported in pancreatic ductal epithelium expressing oncogenic Kras, when challenged by pancreatitis (Lee & Bar-Sagi, 2010). In contrast to the Guerra study (Guerra et al., 2011), oncogenic Kras is shown in the Lee study to suppress pancreatitis-induced premature senescence in ductal epithelium through the Twist-dependent suppression of p16[INK4A] expression (Lee & Bar-Sagi, 2010). The apparent discrepancy between these two studies and the contribution of oncogenic Ras in caerulein-induced senescence may be explained by experimental differences in the stage of the disease (pancreatitis alone vs pancreatitis-induced PDAC) and the cell types (normal ducts vs PanINs) being studied.

2.4 Epigenetic Regulation of the Senescent State in PDAC

Numerous reports point to the establishment, maintenance, and bypass of the senescent state being subject to regulation by epigenetic mechanisms, especially by chromatin modifiers. Senescent cells undergo conformational changes at the chromatin level, giving rise in certain instances to characteristic DNA structures, such as DNA damage foci or SAHFs. In particular, the formation of SAHFs correlates with the recruitment of p16^{INK4A} effector, Rb, along with associated factors heterochromatin protein 1 (HP1), histone methyltransferases (eg, Suv39H1), and histone deacetylases (HDACs), to E2F promoters leading to the silencing of E2F proliferation genes and thereby stabilizing the senescent state (Narita et al., 2003).

In PDAC, most epigenetic mechanisms have been described in the context of senescence bypass. The key senescence effector and tumor suppressor gene *CDKN2A* is almost uniformly inactivated in PDAC patients (Schutte et al., 1997), with 18% of cases resulting from the hypermethylation of its promoter (Ueki et al., 2000). In addition to DNA methylation, *CDKN2A* silencing is also potentially mediated by the Polycomb group (PcG) proteins, transcriptional repressor complexes that silence genes via H3K27 (histone H3 lysine 27 residue) trimethylation (Grzenda, Ordog, & Urrutia, 2011). PcG proteins Bmi1, Ring1b (Martínez-Romero et al., 2009), and Ezh2 (Ougolkov, Bilim, & Billadeau, 2008) are overexpressed in PanINs and PDAC, suggesting that PcG proteins may be mediating senescence bypass via their ability to silence the *CDKN2A* locus. Other epigenetic molecules upregulated in pancreatic cancer include HDACs, such as HDAC2 in undifferentiated PDAC tumors (Fritsche et al., 2009) and HDAC7 in PDAC vs other pancreatic tumor types (Ouaissi et al., 2008), pointing to the potential utility of using HDAC inhibitors.

2.5 Senescence in Pancreatic Stellate Cells

The pancreatic tumor resides in a complex microenvironment called the stroma, a loosely defined entity consisting of fibroblasts, immune cells, blood vessels, secreted cytokines and factors, and extracellular matrix, whose interactions with the tumor cell remain largely unexplored (Neesse et al., 2015). Resident fibroblasts in the stroma, called pancreatic stellate cells (PSCs), have also been described to undergo senescence in vitro, which increases their susceptibility to NK-cell-mediated cytolysis and overlaps with markers of PSC activation in a rat model of acute pancreatitis (Fitzner et al., 2012). While these experiments have been performed in a non-PDAC setting, PSC activation and its protumorigenic role in pancreatic cancer has been extensively reported (Apte et al., 2004; Mace et al., 2013; Vonlaufen et al., 2008), and thus the role of PSC senescence in the context of PSC activation-mediated tumorigenesis in pancreatic cancer is worth exploring.

3. SENESCENCE AND INFLAMMATION IN PANCREATIC CANCER

The link between PDAC and inflammation is well established. First, chronic pancreatitis is an important risk factor of PDAC (Lowenfels et al., 1993). Second, an abundant desmoplastic reaction composed in part of immune cells fundamentally accompanies the disease from inception to invasion. Immune infiltrates at the lesion sites dynamically evolve as the cancer progresses: an early wave of macrophage-enriched infiltration characterizes early grade PanINs, while immunosuppressive populations, such as tumor-associated macrophages (TAM), regulatory T cells, and myeloid-derived suppressor cells (MDSC) soon dominate and persist until the invasive stage (Clark et al., 2007). This latter infiltration of immune cells converts the canonically antitumoral immune microenvironment into a tumor-permissive milieu marked by T-cell suppression and exclusion (Joyce & Fearon, 2015). Key cytokines have been identified that mediate the mobilization of immunosuppressive cells into the PDAC microenvironment: tumor-derived GM-CSF is required for MDSC recruitment (Bayne et al., 2012; Pylayeva-Gupta, Lee, Hajdu, Miller, & Bar-Sagi, 2012); CSF1, overexpressed in PDAC, regulates the TAM phenotype (Zhu et al., 2014); and CXCL12, expressed by a subpopulation of stromal fibroblasts, mediates T-cell exclusion (Feig et al., 2013). All these point to an intimate relationship between the tumor cell and each of the different components of the stromal microenvironment. Recent evidence has shown that senescent cells are capable of influencing their inflammatory microenvironment through the SASP.

3.1 The SASP Links Senescence to Inflammation

In addition to cell cycle exit, senescent cells exhibit specific hallmarks, including the secretion of a discrete set of proinflammatory cytokines, chemokines, growth factors, and matrix-remodeling enzymes collectively referred to as the SASP (Acosta et al., 2013; Coppé et al., 2008; Kuilman et al., 2008). The SASP creates a proinflammatory environment at the tumor site, which is believed to reinforce senescence, and promote immune clearance (Perez-Mancera, Young, & Narita, 2014) (Fig. 1). While mostly protective against tumorigenesis, there is accumulating evidence that a prolonged or deregulated SASP can have tumorigenic functions in the microenvironment (Coppé et al., 2008; Krtolica, Parrinello, Lockett,

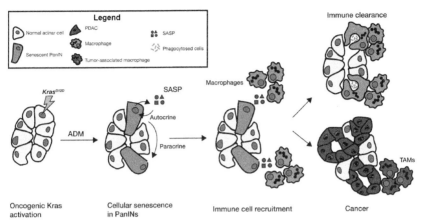

Fig. 1 The dual roles of senescence in pancreatic cancer. Senescent cells, through the SASP, secrete factors and cytokines that attract immune cells to the lesion site. During PDAC progression, upon activation of oncogenic Kras ($Kras^{G12D}$), pancreatic acinar cells undergo acinar–ductal metaplasia (ADM) and develop into preneoplastic lesions called PanINs. A subpopulation of these PanINs undergoes senescence. Through the SASP, senescence could either promote or block tumor progression. Reports in other cancers have pointed to the SASP being responsible for either suppressing tumor formation via immune clearance of senescent cells or driving carcinogenesis via the remodeling of the microenvironment that would favor tumor growth and full-blown cancer. (See the color plate.)

Desprez, & Campisi, 2001) (Fig. 1). In a highly inflammatory cancer like PDAC, the impact of the SASP has not been extensively studied; and thus the noncell autonomous role that senescent cells play in the evolution of the inflammatory tumor microenvironment remains for the most part unknown.

A number of SASP factors have been reported in the context of PDAC. Expression of IL-1α, a SASP component, is believed to serve as the initiating event in the secretion of the SASP by senescent cells (Acosta et al., 2013). Its function in PDAC, while not completely understood, has been suggested by different studies. Indeed, IL-1α is activated downstream of oncogenic Kras, and its overexpression correlates with *KRAS* mutation status and poor survival in human PDAC (Ling et al., 2012). It functions, among other pathways, through NF-κB signaling, a known critical regulator of Ras-driven tumorigenesis (Daniluk et al., 2012). It activates and sustains NF-κB signaling in an autoregulatory loop together with p62 (Ling et al., 2012). Inhibition of IL-1α-induced NF-κB activity by administration of an IL-1 receptor inhibitor halts murine PDAC tumorigenesis, highlighting the therapeutic use of IL-1α inhibition in PDAC (Zhuang et al., 2016). There is some evidence that suggest a SASP-based mechanism of IL-1α function in PDAC. First, NF-κB inhibition leads to the complete abrogation of the SASP in mouse PDAC, which results in the absence of an inflammatory response and improved survival (Ling et al., 2012). Furthermore, abrogation of senescence by inactivation of senescence-associated Sin3B complex in murine PDAC impairs inflammation and correlates with decreased *Il-1α* expression (Rielland et al., 2014). Other SASP factors that have been described in PDAC include IL-6, which is required for Ras tumorigenesis in some PDAC cell lines (Ancrile, Lim, & Counter, 2007), and Tgfβ, the inactivation of which attenuates senescence (Acosta et al., 2013).

3.2 Senescence-Inflammation Interface in PDAC

Through the SASP, senescent cells, whether they comprise tumor or stroma, are capable of altering the inflammatory landscape within the microenvironment, resulting in either pro- or antitumorigenic properties. In PDAC where inflammation represents an early event, senescence and inflammation significantly overlap, not least at inception. Acinar-to-ductal metaplasia (ADM), a process by which acinar cells acquire abnormal tubular structures with ductal parenchyma (Hruban et al., 2006), is believed to be an early event in PDAC, and to precede PanIN formation (Guerra et al., 2007; Zhu, Shi, Schmidt, Hruban, & Konieczny, 2007). ADMs have been described in mouse models of both pancreatitis and acinar promoter-driven PDAC, and also in human pancreata, particularly in those with chronic pancreatitis (Hruban et al., 2006). These ADMs undergo senescence in murine PDAC (Caldwell et al., 2012; Guerra et al., 2007) and express notably higher p21 and p53 than early grade PanINs (Caldwell et al., 2012). However, the relationship between senescent ADMs and inflammation within the context of emerging PDAC is still unclear.

As mentioned earlier, during preinvasive PDAC development, when ADMs are common within the pancreas parenchyma, macrophages generally comprise the first wave of immune infiltrates near PanIN lesions (Clark et al., 2007). They are known to secrete factors including RANTES, TNFα (Liou et al., 2013), and IL-6 (Lesina et al., 2011), which have been shown to promote ADM through NF-κB and STAT3/MMP7 signaling, respectively (Crawford, Scoggins, Washington, Matrisian, & Leach, 2002; Daniluk et al., 2012). Furthermore, recent evidence has shown that ICAM-1, a known SASP factor secreted by oncogenic Kras-expressing acinar cells, promotes the recruitment of these macrophages to sites of ADMs (Liou et al., 2015).

It remains to be determined whether senescence ever plays a role in this process, and whether senescence restricts ADM progression into more developed pancreatic neoplastic lesions (Caldwell et al., 2012).

4. CONCLUSIONS AND SOME UNANSWERED QUESTIONS

PDAC remains a uniformly lethal cancer characterized by a surprisingly long latency (Yachida et al., 2010) and an aggressive, highly metastatic invasive phase. These aspects of its pathobiology make it a difficult disease to manage in the clinic. Based on current data, cellular senescence appears to play dual roles at different stages of PDAC pathogenesis. Despite significant advances in our understanding of the basic biology of PDAC, several questions remain unanswered.

4.1 Oncogenic Kras as Primary Inducer of Senescence in PDAC

Despite the solid body of evidence demonstrating the primary role of oncogenic Kras in the induction of senescence in PDAC, some evidence point to different nuances in this aspect of oncogenic Kras activity. First, while only mutant Kras-expressing cells have been found to be senescent in PDAC, not all mutant Kras-expressing cells become senescent; in fact, only a subpopulation of about 10% of PanIN-1 cells is SA-β-gal-positive (Caldwell et al., 2012). Moreover, in a human autopsy study, *KRAS* mutations and ductal lesions have also been observed in normal pancreata (Luttges et al., 1999). These observations hint at unidentified requirements for mutant Kras to promote senescence, and that, possibly, additional events are required for activated Kras to act as a potent oncogene (Huang et al., 2014). In addition, the observation that mutant Kras exerts a rather inhibitory effect on senescence in pancreatic duct epithelium subjected to pancreatitis (Lee & Bar-Sagi, 2010) suggests that senescence may vary from one cell type to another. Moreover, the possibility that PSCs undergo senescence upon pancreatitis induction (Fitzner et al., 2012) in the absence of oncogenic Kras, suggests that other unidentified cues could also drive certain cells into senescence. This is reminiscent of what has been observed in hepatic stellate cells (Krizhanovsky et al., 2008), but has yet to be investigated in the PDAC context.

4.2 Bidirectional Reversibility of the Senescent State

Senescence was first thought to be an irreversible process; however, reports have later shown that acute somatic inactivation of either Rb (Sage et al.,

2003) or p53 (Beauséjour et al., 2003) can result in senescence bypass. There is intriguing evidence that this bypass can be later reversed, thus reestablishing senescence, for example, upon rapamycin administration (Kennedy et al., 2011) or caerulein treatment cessation (Guerra et al., 2011). Most notably, in an analysis of nine human pancreatitis biopsies, only those (4/9) that have had preoperative exposure to antiinflammatory drugs contained p16^{INK4A}-positive, Ki67-negative low-grade PanINs, indicative of senescence (Guerra et al., 2011). These observations, albeit limited in sample size and in follow-up, point to the fluidity of the senescent state, and the possibility of inducing senescence or its bypass via these yet unclear mechanisms, ultimately modulating cancer progression. While mTOR signaling is clearly involved (Kennedy et al., 2011; Laberge et al., 2015), the molecular mechanism underlying the impact of inflammation on senescence bypass is virtually unknown.

4.3 On the Pro- and Antitumorigenic Roles of Senescence

Another gray area in our understanding of senescence, not only in PDAC, but also in other cancers, is what makes senescence pro- or antitumorigenic. Is it a case of two senescence programs, beneficial or detrimental, or a single good senescence program whose impact is dependent on the context? If the latter is true, the cellular and molecular determinants driving such dichotomy have yet to be elucidated. Are these programs cell type-dependent? What are the physiological contexts in which the same senescent cell could behave differently? In PDAC, a striking observation that begs us to rethink senescence is the presence of p16^{INK4A}-positive PanIN-1 cells in patients with PDAC (Guerra et al., 2011), a stage wherein cancer cells are generally believed to have had bypassed senescence. In liver cancer, senescent hepatic stellate cells have been described to be either beneficial in resolving fibrosis (Krizhanovsky et al., 2008) or tumor-promoting through the SASP (Yoshimoto et al., 2013). Similarly, there is a need to understand the role of senescent cells during more advanced stages of PDAC, their effect on other cells in the same microenvironment (and if there actually are other senescent cell types), and their net effect on tumorigenesis.

4.4 Senescent Cell-Immune Cell Interactions

In PDAC, senescence and inflammation clearly overlap, and it has recently been suggested that the SASP may represent one of the molecular links between these processes (Fig. 1). This observation raises more questions:

how does the SASP vary through time, and accordingly, how does the SASP influence the inflammatory repertoire in the presence of the ongoing infiltration that accompanies PDAC development? What does the SASP of senescent PanIN-1 cells consist of? A possible scenario that could help explain why few senescent cells are being detected is that most senescent cells may be constantly getting cleared by immune cells (Hoenicke & Zender, 2012) (Fig. 1), which are known to infiltrate the parenchyma during the earliest phases (Clark et al., 2007). However, immune clearance remains to be investigated during any stage of PDAC progression.

Taken all together, studies on cellular senescence have revealed important insights into PDAC pathogenesis, especially during its earliest stages, when senescence is known to first occur. However, several issues related to the field of senescence as it relates to tumorigenesis remain to be addressed, in addition to the unanswered questions mentioned before: first, can we positively identify senescence in vivo, and are all senescent cells created equal based on their autocrine and paracrine properties (Sharpless & Sherr, 2015)?; second, what is the fate of senescent cells during cancer progression?; and finally, can we expand the vast and invaluable knowledge acquired in the past using mouse models to human tumors (McDonald et al., 2012)?

ACKNOWLEDGMENTS

We would like to thank all the members of the David Laboratory for helpful discussions. Work in the David laboratory is funded by the National Institute of Health (5R01CA148639 and 5R21CA155736 to G.D.), the Irma T. Hirschl Charitable Trust (G.D.), the Samuel Waxman Cancer Research Foundation (G.D.), and a Feinberg NYU individual grant (G.D.).

REFERENCES

Acosta, J. C., Banito, A., Wuestefeld, T., Georgilis, A., Janich, P., Morton, J. P., et al. (2013). A complex secretory program orchestrated by the inflammasome controls paracrine senescence. *Nature Cell Biology*, *15*, 978–990.

Aguirre, A. J., Bardeesy, N., Sinha, M., Lopez, L., Tuveson, D. A., Horner, J., et al. (2003). Activated Kras and Ink4a/Arf deficiency cooperate to produce metastatic pancreatic ductal adenocarcinoma. *Genes & Development*, *17*, 3112–3126.

Ancrile, B., Lim, K.-H., & Counter, C. M. (2007). Oncogenic Ras-induced secretion of IL6 is required for tumorigenesis. *Genes & Development*, *21*, 1714–1719.

Apte, M. V., Park, S., Phillips, P. A., Santucci, N., Goldstein, D., Kumar, R. K., et al. (2004). Desmoplastic reaction in pancreatic cancer: Role of pancreatic stellate cells. *Pancreas*, *29*, 179–187.

Bardeesy, N., Aguirre, A. J., Chu, G. C., Cheng, K.-H., Lopez, L. V., Hezel, A. F., et al. (2006). Both p16(Ink4a) and the p19(Arf)-p53 pathway constrain progression of pancreatic adenocarcinoma in the mouse. *Proceedings of the National Academy of Sciences of the United States of America*, *103*, 5947–5952.

Bayne, L. J., Beatty, G. L., Jhala, N., Clark, C. E., Rhim, A. D., Stanger, B. Z., et al. (2012). Tumor-derived granulocyte-macrophage colony-stimulating factor regulates myeloid inflammation and T cell immunity in pancreatic cancer. *Cancer Cell, 21*, 822–835.

Beauséjour, C. M., Krtolica, A., Galimi, F., Narita, M., Lowe, S. W., Yaswen, P., et al. (2003). Reversal of human cellular senescence: Roles of the p53 and p16 pathways. *The EMBO Journal, 22*, 4212–4222.

Caldwell, M. E., DeNicola, G. M., Martins, C. P., Jacobetz, M. A., Maitra, A., Hruban, R. H., et al. (2012). Cellular features of senescence during the evolution of human and murine ductal pancreatic cancer. *Oncogene, 31*, 1599–1608.

Carrière, C., Gore, A. J., Norris, A. M., Gunn, J. R., Young, A. L., Longnecker, D. S., et al. (2011). Deletion of Rb accelerates pancreatic carcinogenesis by oncogenic Kras and impairs senescence in premalignant lesions. *Gastroenterology, 141*, 1091–1101.

Clark, C. E., Hingorani, S. R., Mick, R., Combs, C., Tuveson, D. A., & Vonderheide, R. H. (2007). Dynamics of the immune reaction to pancreatic cancer from inception to invasion. *Cancer Research, 67*, 9518–9527.

Collado, M., Gil, J., Efeyan, A., Guerra, C., Schuhmacher, A. J., Barradas, M., et al. (2005). Tumour biology: Senescence in premalignant tumours. *Nature, 436*, 642.

Collado, M., & Serrano, M. (2010). Senescence in tumours: Evidence from mice and humans. *Nature Reviews. Cancer, 10*, 51–57.

Coppé, J.-P., Desprez, P.-Y., Krtolica, A., & Campisi, J. (2010). The senescence-associated secretory phenotype: The dark side of tumor suppression. *Annual Review of Pathology, 5*, 99–118.

Coppé, J.-P., Patil, C. K., Rodier, F., Sun, Y., Muñoz, D. P., Goldstein, J., et al. (2008). Senescence-associated secretory phenotypes reveal cell-nonautonomous functions of oncogenic RAS and the p53 tumor suppressor. *PLoS Biology, 6*, 2853–2868.

Crawford, H. C., Scoggins, C. R., Washington, M. K., Matrisian, L. M., & Leach, S. D. (2002). Matrix metalloproteinase-7 is expressed by pancreatic cancer precursors and regulates acinar-to-ductal metaplasia in exocrine pancreas. *The Journal of Clinical Investigation, 109*, 1437–1444.

Daniluk, J., Liu, Y., Deng, D., Chu, J., Huang, H., Gaiser, S., et al. (2012). An NF-κB pathway-mediated positive feedback loop amplifies Ras activity to pathological levels in mice. *The Journal of Clinical Investigation, 122*, 1519–1528.

Di Micco, R., Fumagalli, M., Cicalese, A., Piccinin, S., Gasparini, P., Luise, C., et al. (2006). Oncogene-induced senescence is a DNA damage response triggered by DNA hyper-replication. *Nature, 444*, 638–642.

Dimri, G. P., Lee, X., Basile, G., Acosta, M., Scott, G., Roskelley, C., et al. (1995). A biomarker that identifies senescent human cells in culture and in aging skin in vivo. *Proceedings of the National Academy of Sciences of the United States of America, 92*, 9363–9367.

Eser, S., Reiff, N., Messer, M., Seidler, B., Gottschalk, K., Dobler, M., et al. (2013). Selective requirement of PI3K/PDK1 signaling for Kras oncogene-driven pancreatic cell plasticity and cancer. *Cancer Cell, 23*, 406–420.

Feig, C., Jones, J. O., Kraman, M., Wells, R. J., Deonarine, A., Chan, D. S., et al. (2013). Targeting CXCL12 from FAP-expressing carcinoma-associated fibroblasts synergizes with anti-PD-L1 immunotherapy in pancreatic cancer. *Proceedings of the National Academy of Sciences of the United States of America, 110*, 20212–20217.

Feldmann, G., Beaty, R., Hruban, R. H., & Maitra, A. (2007). Molecular genetics of pancreatic intraepithelial neoplasia. *Journal of Hepato-Biliary-Pancreatic Surgery, 14*, 224–232.

Fitzner, B., Müller, S., Walther, M., Fischer, M., Engelmann, R., Müller-Hilke, B., et al. (2012). Senescence determines the fate of activated rat pancreatic stellate cells. *Journal of Cellular and Molecular Medicine, 16*, 2620–2630.

Fritsche, P., Seidler, B., Schuler, S., Schnieke, A., Gottlicher, M., Schmid, R. M., et al. (2009). HDAC2 mediates therapeutic resistance of pancreatic cancer cells via the BH3-only protein NOXA. *Gut*, *58*, 1399–1409.

Grzenda, A., Ordog, T., & Urrutia, R. (2011). Polycomb and the emerging epigenetics of pancreatic cancer. *Journal of Gastrointestinal Cancer*, *42*, 100–111.

Guerra, C., Collado, M., Navas, C., Schuhmacher, A. J., Hernández-Porras, I., Cañamero, M., et al. (2011). Pancreatitis-induced inflammation contributes to pancreatic cancer by inhibiting oncogene-induced senescence. *Cancer Cell*, *19*, 728–739.

Guerra, C., Schuhmacher, A. J., Cañamero, M., Grippo, P. J., Verdaguer, L., Pérez-Gallego, L., et al. (2007). Chronic pancreatitis is essential for induction of pancreatic ductal adenocarcinoma by K-Ras oncogenes in adult mice. *Cancer Cell*, *11*, 291–302.

Hingorani, S. R., Petricoin, E. F., Maitra, A., Rajapakse, V., King, C., Jacobetz, M. A., et al. (2003). Preinvasive and invasive ductal pancreatic cancer and its early detection in the mouse. *Cancer Cell*, *4*, 437–450.

Hingorani, S. R., Wang, L., Multani, A. S., Combs, C., Deramaudt, T. B., Hruban, R. H., et al. (2005). Trp53R172H and KrasG12D cooperate to promote chromosomal instability and widely metastatic pancreatic ductal adenocarcinoma in mice. *Cancer Cell*, *7*, 469–483.

Hoenicke, L., & Zender, L. (2012). Immune surveillance of senescent cells—Biological significance in cancer- and non-cancer pathologies. *Carcinogenesis*, *33*, 1123–1126.

Hruban, R. H., Adsay, N. V., Albores-Saavedra, J., Anver, M. R., Biankin, A. V., Boivin, G. P., et al. (2006). Pathology of genetically engineered mouse models of pancreatic exocrine cancer: Consensus report and recommendations. *Cancer Research*, *66*, 95–106.

Hruban, R. H., Goggins, M., Parsons, J., & Kern, S. E. (2000). Progression model for pancreatic cancer. *Clinical Cancer Research*, *6*, 2969–2972.

Hruban, R. H., Takaori, K., Klimstra, D. S., Adsay, N. V., Albores-Saavedra, J., Biankin, A. V., et al. (2004). An illustrated consensus on the classification of pancreatic intraepithelial neoplasia and intraductal papillary mucinous neoplasms. *The American Journal of Surgical Pathology*, *28*, 977–987.

Huang, H., Daniluk, J., Liu, Y., Chu, J., Li, Z., Ji, B., et al. (2014). Oncogenic K-Ras requires activation for enhanced activity. *Oncogene*, *33*, 532–535.

Iannello, A., Thompson, T. W., Ardolino, M., Lowe, S. W., & Raulet, D. H. (2013). p53-dependent chemokine production by senescent tumor cells supports NKG2D-dependent tumor elimination by natural killer cells. *The Journal of Experimental Medicine*, *210*, 2057–2069.

Ijichi, H., Chytil, A., Gorska, A. E., Aakre, M. E., Fujitani, Y., Fujitani, S., et al. (2006). Aggressive pancreatic ductal adenocarcinoma in mice caused by pancreas-specific blockade of transforming growth factor-beta signaling in cooperation with active Kras expression. *Genes & Development*, *20*, 3147–3160.

Joyce, J. A., & Fearon, D. T. (2015). T cell exclusion, immune privilege, and the tumor microenvironment. *Science*, *348*, 74–80.

Kang, T.-W., Yevsa, T., Woller, N., Hoenicke, L., Wuestefeld, T., Dauch, D., et al. (2011). Senescence surveillance of pre-malignant hepatocytes limits liver cancer development. *Nature*, *479*, 547–551.

Kennedy, A. L., Morton, J. P., Manoharan, I., Nelson, D. M., Jamieson, N. B., Pawlikowski, J. S., et al. (2011). Activation of the PIK3CA/AKT pathway suppresses senescence induced by an activated RAS oncogene to promote tumorigenesis. *Molecular Cell*, *42*, 36–49.

Krizhanovsky, V., Yon, M., Dickins, R. A., Hearn, S., Simon, J., Miething, C., et al. (2008). Senescence of activated stellate cells limits liver fibrosis. *Cell*, *134*, 657–667.

Krtolica, A., Parrinello, S., Lockett, S., Desprez, P. Y., & Campisi, J. (2001). Senescent fibroblasts promote epithelial cell growth and tumorigenesis: A link between cancer and aging. *Proceedings of the National Academy of Sciences of the United States of America*, *98*, 12072–12077.

Kuilman, T., Michaloglou, C., Mooi, W. J., & Peeper, D. S. (2010). The essence of senescence. *Genes & Development*, *24*, 2463–2479.

Kuilman, T., Michaloglou, C., Vredeveld, L. C. W., Douma, S., van Doorn, R., Desmet, C. J., et al. (2008). Oncogene-induced senescence relayed by an interleukin-dependent inflammatory network. *Cell*, *133*, 1019–1031.

Kurz, D. J., Decary, S., Hong, Y., & Erusalimsky, J. D. (2000). Senescence-associated (beta)-galactosidase reflects an increase in lysosomal mass during replicative ageing of human endothelial cells. *Journal of Cell Science*, *113*(Pt. 20), 3613–3622.

Laberge, R. M., Sun, Y., Orjalo, A. V., Patil, C. K., Freund, A., Zhou, L., et al. (2015). MTOR regulates the pro-tumorigenic senescence-associated secretory phenotype by promoting IL1A translation. *Nature Cell Biology*, *17*, 1049–1061.

Lee, K. E., & Bar-Sagi, D. (2010). Oncogenic KRas suppresses inflammation-associated senescence of pancreatic ductal cells. *Cancer Cell*, *18*, 448–458.

Lesina, M., Kurkowski, M. U., Ludes, K., Rose-John, S., Treiber, M., Klöppel, G., et al. (2011). Stat3/Socs3 activation by IL-6 transsignaling promotes progression of pancreatic intraepithelial neoplasia and development of pancreatic cancer. *Cancer Cell*, *19*, 456–469.

Ling, J., Kang, Y. A., Zhao, R., Xia, Q., Lee, D.-F., Chang, Z., et al. (2012). KrasG12D-induced IKK2/β/NF-κB activation by IL-1α and p62 feedforward loops is required for development of pancreatic ductal adenocarcinoma. *Cancer Cell*, *21*, 105–120.

Liou, G.-Y., Döppler, H., Necela, B., Edenfield, B., Zhang, L., Dawson, D. W., et al. (2015). Mutant KRAS-induced expression of ICAM-1 in pancreatic acinar cells causes attraction of macrophages to expedite the formation of precancerous lesions. *Cancer Discovery*, *5*, 52–63.

Liou, G.-Y., Döppler, H., Necela, B., Krishna, M., Crawford, H. C., Raimondo, M., et al. (2013). Macrophage-secreted cytokines drive pancreatic acinar-to-ductal metaplasia through NF-κB and MMPs. *The Journal of Cell Biology*, *202*, 563–577.

Lowenfels, A. B., Maisonneuve, P., Cavallini, G., Ammann, R. W., Lankisch, P. G., Andersen, J. R., et al. (1993). Pancreatitis and the risk of pancreatic cancer. International Pancreatitis Study Group. *The New England Journal of Medicine*, *328*, 1433–1437.

Luttges, J., Reinecke-Luthge, A., Mollmann, B., Menke, M. A., Clemens, A., Klimpfinger, M., et al. (1999). Duct changes and K-ras mutations in the disease-free pancreas: Analysis of type, age relation and spatial distribution. *Virchows Archiv*, *435*, 461–468.

Mace, T. A., Ameen, Z., Collins, A., Wojcik, S., Mair, M., Young, G. S., et al. (2013). Pancreatic cancer-associated stellate cells promote differentiation of myeloid-derived suppressor cells in a STAT3-dependent manner. *Cancer Research*, *73*, 3007–3018.

Martínez-Romero, C., Rooman, I., Skoudy, A., Guerra, C., Molero, X., González, A., et al. (2009). The epigenetic regulators Bmi1 and Ring1B are differentially regulated in pancreatitis and pancreatic ductal adenocarcinoma. *The Journal of Pathology*, *219*, 205–213.

McDonald, O. G., Maitra, A., & Hruban, R. H. (2012). Human correlates of provocative questions in pancreatic pathology. *Advances in Anatomic Pathology*, *19*, 351–362.

Morton, J. P., Jamieson, N. B., Karim, S. A., Athineos, D., Ridgway, R. A., Nixon, C., et al. (2010). LKB1 haploinsufficiency cooperates with Kras to promote pancreatic cancer through suppression of p21-dependent growth arrest. *Gastroenterology*, *139*, 586–597. 597.e581–586.

Morton, J. P., Timpson, P., Karim, S. A., Ridgway, R. A., Athineos, D., Doyle, B., et al. (2010). Mutant p53 drives metastasis and overcomes growth arrest/senescence in pancreatic cancer. *Proceedings of the National Academy of Sciences of the United States of America*, *107*, 246–251.

Muñoz-Espín, D., & Serrano, M. (2014). Cellular senescence: From physiology to pathology. *Nature Reviews. Molecular Cell Biology, 15*, 482–496.

Narita, M., Núñez, S., Heard, E., Narita, M., Lin, A. W., Hearn, S. A., et al. (2003). Rb-mediated heterochromatin formation and silencing of E2F target genes during cellular senescence. *Cell, 113*, 703–716.

Neesse, A., Algul, H., Tuveson, D. A., & Gress, T. M. (2015). Stromal biology and therapy in pancreatic cancer: A changing paradigm. *Gut, 64*, 1476–1484.

Ouaissi, M., Sielezneff, I., Silvestre, R., Sastre, B., Bernard, J. P., Lafontaine, J. S., et al. (2008). High histone deacetylase 7 (HDAC7) expression is significantly associated with adenocarcinomas of the pancreas. *Annals of Surgical Oncology, 15*, 2318–2328.

Ougolkov, A. V., Bilim, V. N., & Billadeau, D. D. (2008). Regulation of pancreatic tumor cell proliferation and chemoresistance by the histone methyltransferase enhancer of zeste homologue 2. *Clinical Cancer Research, 14*, 6790–6796.

Pérez-Mancera, P. A., Guerra, C., Barbacid, M., & Tuveson, D. A. (2012). What we have learned about pancreatic cancer from mouse models. *Gastroenterology, 142*, 1079–1092.

Perez-Mancera, P. A., Young, A. R., & Narita, M. (2014). Inside and out: The activities of senescence in cancer. *Nature Reviews. Cancer, 14*, 547–558.

Pylayeva-Gupta, Y., Lee, K. E., Hajdu, C. H., Miller, G., & Bar-Sagi, D. (2012). Oncogenic Kras-induced GM-CSF production promotes the development of pancreatic neoplasia. *Cancer Cell, 21*, 836–847.

Rielland, M., Cantor, D. J., Graveline, R., Hajdu, C., Mara, L., Diaz Bde, D., et al. (2014). Senescence-associated SIN3B promotes inflammation and pancreatic cancer progression. *The Journal of Clinical Investigation, 124*, 2125–2135.

Ryan, D. P., Hong, T. S., & Bardeesy, N. (2014). Pancreatic adenocarcinoma. *The New England Journal of Medicine, 371*, 1039–1049.

Sage, J., Miller, A. L., Perez-Mancera, P. A., Wysocki, J. M., & Jacks, T. (2003). Acute mutation of retinoblastoma gene function is sufficient for cell cycle re-entry. *Nature, 424*, 223–228.

Schutte, M., Hruban, R. H., Geradts, J., Maynard, R., Hilgers, W., Rabindran, S. K., et al. (1997). Abrogation of the Rb/p16 tumor-suppressive pathway in virtually all pancreatic carcinomas. *Cancer Research, 57*, 3126–3130.

Serrano, M., Hannon, G. J., & Beach, D. (1993). A new regulatory motif in cell-cycle control causing specific inhibition of cyclin D/CDK4. *Nature, 366*, 704–707.

Sharpless, N. E., & Sherr, C. J. (2015). Forging a signature of in vivo senescence. *Nature Reviews. Cancer, 15*, 397–408.

Shi, C., Hong, S.-M., Lim, P., Kamiyama, H., Khan, M., Anders, R. A., et al. (2009). KRAS2 mutations in human pancreatic acinar-ductal metaplastic lesions are limited to those with PanIN: Implications for the human pancreatic cancer cell of origin. *Molecular Cancer Research, 7*, 230–236.

Siegel, R. L., Miller, K. D., & Jemal, A. (2016). Cancer statistics, 2016. *CA: A Cancer Journal for Clinicians, 66*, 7–30.

Ueki, T., Toyota, M., Sohn, T., Yeo, C. J., Issa, J. P., Hruban, R. H., et al. (2000). Hypermethylation of multiple genes in pancreatic adenocarcinoma. *Cancer Research, 60*, 1835–1839.

van Heek, N. T., Meeker, A. K., Kern, S. E., Yeo, C. J., Lillemoe, K. D., Cameron, J. L., et al. (2002). Telomere shortening is nearly universal in pancreatic intraepithelial neoplasia. *The American Journal of Pathology, 161*, 1541–1547.

Vonlaufen, A., Joshi, S., Qu, C., Phillips, P. A., Xu, Z., Parker, N. R., et al. (2008). Pancreatic stellate cells: Partners in crime with pancreatic cancer cells. *Cancer Research, 68*, 2085–2093.

Xue, W., Zender, L., Miething, C., Dickins, R. A., Hernando, E., Krizhanovsky, V., et al. (2007). Senescence and tumour clearance is triggered by p53 restoration in murine liver carcinomas. *Nature, 445*, 656–660.

Yachida, S., Jones, S., Bozic, I., Antal, T., Leary, R., Fu, B., et al. (2010). Distant metastasis occurs late during the genetic evolution of pancreatic cancer. *Nature*, *467*, 1114–1117.

Yoshimoto, S., Lqo, T. M., Atarashi, K., Kanda, H., Sato, S., Oyadomari, S., et al. (2013). Obesity-induced gut microbial metabolite promotes liver cancer through senescence secretome. *Nature*, *499*, 97–101.

Zhu, Y., Knolhoff, B. L., Meyer, M. A., Nywening, T. M., West, B. L., Luo, J., et al. (2014). CSF1/CSF1R blockade reprograms tumor-infiltrating macrophages and improves response to T-cell checkpoint immunotherapy in pancreatic cancer models. *Cancer Research*, *74*, 5057–5069.

Zhu, L., Shi, G., Schmidt, C. M., Hruban, R. H., & Konieczny, S. F. (2007). Acinar cells contribute to the molecular heterogeneity of pancreatic intraepithelial neoplasia. *The American Journal of Pathology*, *171*, 263–273.

Zhuang, Z., Ju, H. Q., Aguilar, M., Gocho, T., Li, H., Iida, T., et al. (2016). IL1 receptor antagonist inhibits pancreatic cancer growth by abrogating NF-kappaB activation. *Clinical Cancer Research*, *22*, 1432–1444.

CHAPTER TWO

Small-Molecule Targeting of BET Proteins in Cancer

C.A. French[1]

Brigham and Women's Hospital, Harvard Medical School, Boston, MA, United States
[1]Corresponding author: e-mail address: cfrench@partners.org

Contents

Abstract

BET proteins have recently become recognized for their role in a broad range of cancers and are defined by the presence of two acetyl-histone reading bromodomains and an ET domain. This family of proteins includes BRD2, BRD3, BRD4, and BRDT. BRD4 is the most-studied BET protein in cancer, and normally serves as an epigenetic reader that links active chromatin marks to transcriptional elongation through activation of RNA polymerase II. The role of BRD3 and BRD4 first became known in cancer as mutant oncoproteins fused to the p300-recruiting NUT protein in a rare aggressive subtype of squamous cell cancer known as NUT midline carcinoma (NMC). BET inhibitors are

Advances in Cancer Research, Volume 131
ISSN 0065-230X
http://dx.doi.org/10.1016/bs.acr.2016.04.001

acetyl-histone mimetics that specifically bind BET bromodomains, competitively inhibiting its engagement with chromatin. The antineoplastic effects of BET inhibitors were first demonstrated in NMC and have since been shown to be effective at inhibiting the growth of many different cancers, particularly acute leukemia. BET inhibitors have also been instrumental as tool compounds that have demonstrated the key role of BRD4 in driving NMC and non-NMC cancer growth. Many clinical trials enrolling patients with hematologic and solid tumors are ongoing, with encouraging preliminary findings. BET proteins BRD2, BRD3, and BRD4 are expressed in nearly all cells of the body, so there are concerns of toxicity with BET inhibitors, as well as the development of resistance. Toxicity and resistance may be overcome by combining BET inhibitors with other targeted inhibitors, or through the use of novel BET inhibitor derivatives.

1. INTRODUCTION

Cancer arises from gene mutation and ultimately involves aberrant epigenetic chromatin regulation. Chromatin, comprised of DNA, nucleosomes, and associated transcription factors, can be either transcriptionally active or inactive, as defined in part by epigenetic posttranslational modifications of histone tails. An active chromatin state is associated with acetylated histones that, through their negative electric charge, decrease the interaction between the positively charged histone N-termini with the negatively charged phosphate groups of DNA. This process of acetylation thus relaxes chromatin, making it accessible to transcriptional machinery. The epigenetic state of chromatin must be decoded for the regulation of gene expression. This encoding and decoding of chromatin is accomplished through the action of so-called chromatin "readers," "writers," and "erasers," and cancer can occur through abnormalities of any one or more of these factors. Histone acetyltransferases (HATs) and methyltransferases are typical epigenetic writers that transfer acetyl or methyl groups onto histone tails. Histone deacetylases (HDAC) and demethylases are erasers that remove these marks. Bromodomains are protein modules that recognize and read acetyl–histone marks associated with open active chromatin and are present within a large number of proteins, including HATs. Proteins that contain two bromodomains and an extraterminal (ET) protein–protein interaction motif are readers of the BET family. Examples of aberrant chromatin modifiers in cancer include chromosomal rearrangements of the histone methyl transferase, *MLL*, and of the *CBP* HAT writers in acute leukemia (Dash & Gilliland, 2001; Muntean & Hess, 2012). Overexpression or enhanced activity of the polycomb component EZH2 histone methyltransferase (HMT) has been correlated with the aggressiveness of a number of solid tumors, including, breast and prostate cancer (Chase & Cross, 2011; Deb, Thakur, & Gupta, 2013). Finally, fusion of the BET reader encoding gene, *BRD3* or *BRD4*, to *nuclear protein in testis* (*NUT*) is the driving genetic event in NUT midline carcinoma (NMC) (French et al., 2003, 2008). Therapeutic targeting of chromatin modifier proteins in cancer has been challenging due to the ubiquitous role these proteins play in normal healthy cells. For example, HDAC inhibitors can be effective anticancer reagents, but are limited by toxicity due to a broad range of effects on normal cell physiologic processes. Over the past 5 years BET inhibitors targeting BET proteins have emerged as a potentially more tolerable therapy that may specifically inhibit the expression of key cancer-associated genes. Why they appear to more specifically inhibit cancer gene expression is not completely understood, but is the subject of intense investigation. This review will focus on the aberrant BET protein readers in cancer and how they are being targeted using novel small molecules. Particular consideration will be made to the pathogenesis of the paradigmatic cancer harboring, the only known oncoprotein form of BRD4/BRD3, NMC, and how this pathway is targeted by BET inhibitors.

2. BET PROTEINS
2.1 The Bromodomain

The bromodomain consists of four alpha helices connected by variable loops that collectively form a hydrophobic pocket (Dhalluin et al., 1999). The hydrophobic pocket recognizes acetylated lysine tails of histones and other proteins; thus, the reading function of bromodomains is not restricted to nucleosomes, but can interact with a much larger range of proteins (Dhalluin et al., 1999). There are 46 different human bromodomain-containing proteins (Chaidos, Caputo, & Karadimitris, 2015) consisting of HATs, methyltransferases, helicases, chromatin remodelers, transcriptional coactivators/mediators, and BET proteins (Filippakopoulos & Knapp, 2012; Filippakopoulos et al., 2012). Bromodomain specificity is determined by the amino acid sequence within the binding pocket (Filippakopoulos et al., 2012). BET proteins recognize acetylated histone H3 and H4 residues (Dey, Chitsaz, Abbasi, Misteli, & Ozato, 2003), and with greater affinity for multiple acetylations present within a span of 1–5 amino acids (Filippakopoulos et al., 2012).

2.2 BET Function

The BET protein family consists of BRD2, BRD3, BRD4, and BRDT. BRD2–4 are ubiquitously expressed, whereas BRDT expression is restricted to the testis (Pivot-Pajot et al., 2003). The first described BET encoding gene was the female sterile homeotic (*fs*(*1*)*h*) in *Drosophila* (Digan et al., 1986), and the first mammalian BET protein functionally characterized was BRD2 (Denis & Green, 1996). BRD2 functions to recognize acetyl-lysines, particularly histone H4, and acts as a protein scaffold to regulate and enable transcription (Crowley, Kaine, Yoshida, Nandi, & Wolgemuth, 2002; Denis, Vaziri, Guo, & Faller, 2000; Denis et al., 2006; Kanno et al., 2004; LeRoy, Rickards, & Flint, 2008; Nakamura et al., 2007). Similarly, BRD4, which has an 80% identical amino acid sequence to that of BRD2, also regulates transcription (Fig. 1). The profound biologic importance of BRD2 and BRD4 is evidenced by the observation that homozygous deletion of either is embryonic lethal (Gyuris et al.,

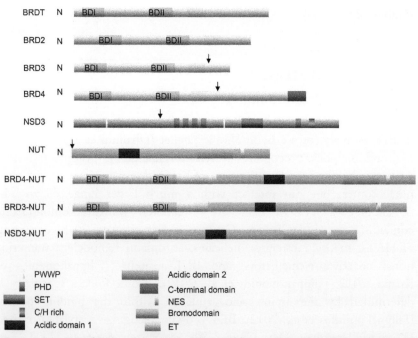

Fig. 1 Schematic of BET proteins, NUT, NSD3, and fusion oncoproteins identified in NUT midline carcinoma (NMC). NUT-fusion breakpoints are indicated by an *arrow*. Neither BRDT nor BRD2 have been involved in a fusion with NUT. (See the color plate.)

2009; Houzelstein et al., 2002; Shang, Wang, Wen, Greenberg, & Wolgemuth, 2009; Wang et al., 2010).

BRD4 was initially described in mice as mitotic chromosome associated protein (Dey et al., 2000), because it remains bound to chromosomes during mitosis, unlike most nuclear proteins, which are evicted during this phase of the cell cycle. Human BRD4, originally termed "HUNK1," was first recognized for its role, as a translocation fusion to the *NUT* gene (Fig. 1), in NMC (French et al., 2001, 2003). The association of BRD4 to acetylated chromatin throughout the cell cycle has led investigators to propose that it bookmarks active genes prior to mitosis for reactivation during G1 (Dey et al., 2000), providing the cell memory of its identity. Indeed, BRD4 is essential for transcription of early M/G1 transition genes, such as *RAN* and *TGIF1*, that are programmed to be expressed at the end of mitosis and beginning of G1 (Dey, Nishiyama, Karpova, McNally, & Ozato, 2009).

Over the past decade and a half, much has been learned of the role of BRD4 in transcription. BRD4 is required for transcriptional elongation. Throughout the genome, thousands of genes are poised for transcription with RNA polymerase II (RNA pol II) adjacent to their transcriptional start sites, but not producing full-length transcripts (Kwak & Lis, 2013). This paused state is released upon engagement of BRD4 with acetyl-histones located at the transcriptional start site (Fig. 2). BRD4, when bound to active acetylated chromatin, is brought in proximity to RNA pol II through its inclusion in the Mediator complex. Mediator, a complex of multiple proteins, links transcription factors to Pol II activation (Jiang et al., 1998). Once docked to active chromatin, BRD4 replaces the repressive HEXIM1/7SK

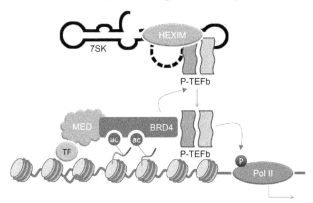

Fig. 2 Mechanism by which BRD4 facilitates transcriptional elongation. (See the color plate.)

snRNP bound to the transcription elongation factor b CyclinT1/CDK9 heterodimer (P-TEFb) (Jang et al., 2005; Yang et al., 2005), by binding P-TEFb with its C-terminal domain (CTD) and second bromodomain (BD2) (Bisgrove, Mahmoudi, Henklein, & Verdin, 2007; Jang et al., 2005; Schroder et al., 2012). Once displaced from HEXIM1/7SK RNA, BRD4-bound P-TEFb phosphorylates RNA pol II at serine 2 to convert it into its actively elongating state (Jang et al., 2005; Yang et al., 2005). Hence, BRD4 is considered essential for the transcription of thousands of genes.

The BRD4 bromodomains do not only bind acetylated histones. They have been shown to interact with acetylated lysine residues of a variety of other proteins, including transcription factors (TFs). Recently, Roe, Mercan, Rivera, Pappin, and Vakoc (2015) demonstrated that BRD4 can bind TF-defined genomic loci. In this study, TFs acetylated by p300 recruited and bound BRD4 to specific loci with which they localized. The findings explain one mechanism by which BRD4 can be recruited to DNA-sequence specific loci, and may help explain how BET inhibitors can have precise inhibitory effects on cancer-specific gene expression.

In additional work done by Wu, Lee, Lai, Zhang, and Chiang (2013), it was found that BRD4 can bind TFs independent of the bromodomain–acetyl-lysine interaction. In this study, BRD4 bound bacterially expressed (thus lacking any posttranslational modifications, such as acetylation) purified Myc/Max heterodimer, p53, YY1, C/EBPα, C/EBPβ, c-Jun, and AP2. In particular, the p53 interaction was mediated by phosphorylation of BRD4 by casein kinase II. Phosphorylation of BRD4 led to conversion of a non-DNA bound to a DNA-bound p53–BRD4 complex, demonstrating a novel mechanism by which BRD4 can regulate TF-specific gene transcription through kinase signaling.

The ET domain of BET proteins serves as a protein interaction module that binds a range of chromatin-modifying proteins, including the transcriptional activating methyltransferase, NSD3, and the arginine demethylase, JMJD6. The functional importance of the NSD3–BRD4 interaction was first shown in NMC, a variant of which harbors a NSD3–NUT-fusion that can completely rescue loss of BRD4–NUT in BRD4–NUT+ NMC (French et al., 2014). Interestingly, only the N-terminus of NSD3, lacking the methyltransferase domain, is part of this fusion (Fig. 1), suggesting that NSD3 may serve primarily as a means to link NUT to BRD4. In line with this oncogenic role of NSD3 an enzymatically inert "molecular glue," recent work by Shen et al. has demonstrated that only a short isoform of

NSD3, lacking its methyltransferase domain, binds to BRD4 and links it to CHD8, a helicase chromatin remodeler (Shen et al., 2015). The functional importance of this interaction has only been demonstrated in a leukemia model, and so it is not known whether this is a normal or exclusively onco-genic function of NSD3 and the ET domain of BRD4. The ET domain also associates with ATP-dependent chromatin remodeling enzymes including the helicase, CHD4, and SMARCA4, a member of the SWI/SNF complex (Rahman et al., 2011). The binding of these factors by ET suggests a yet-to-be understood role of BRD4 in chromatin remodeling. One such role of BRD4-associated remodeling may be to regulate the DNA damage response to irradiation. The recruitment by a novel BRD4 isoform of the condensin II chromatin remodeling complex to acetylated chromatin inhibits DNA damage signaling and repair (Floyd et al., 2013). Insulation by this isoform of BRD4 is associated with an overall more compact chromatin configura-tion, suggesting that its recruitment of condensin II may in fact remodel chromatin. It is unclear whether the interaction with condensin II compo-nents is through the ET or other BRD4 domains, nevertheless this function of BRD4 may have important implications in treatment of patients with BRD4 inhibitors while receiving radiation therapy.

2.3 BETs in Health and Disease

BRD2, BRD3, and BRD4 play key roles in transcription of genes required for both inflammation and cancer. In macrophages, these BET proteins are important proinflammatory transcriptional activators of lipopolysaccha-ride (LPS) induced genes, including IL-1β, IL-6, IL-12α, CXCL9, and CCL12 (Belkina, Nikolajczyk, & Denis, 2013; Hargreaves, Horng, & Medzhitov, 2009; Nicodeme et al., 2010). In fact, inhibition of BET proteins with BET bromodomain inhibitors (described later) can prevent bacterial LPS-induced septic shock in mice through the inhibition of tran-scription of these genes, most notably IL-6, in macrophages (Nicodeme et al., 2010). Work done in BRD2-deficient genetically engineered mice (Denis, 2010; Wang et al., 2010) has shown that BRD2 may be impor-tant in coupling toll-like receptor and TNF signaling to NF-kB-induced transcription of inflammatory genes. In these studies, BRD2 hypomorphic mice lack inflammation-associated, obesity-induced insulin resistance. Finally, there is evidence that BET proteins may also play a role in T helper cell-mediated autoimmune disease (Bandukwala et al., 2012; Mele et al., 2013).

In addition to its role in inflammation, BRD4 plays important roles in viral biology. In HIV infection, BRD4 competes with HIV TAT protein for interaction with PTEF-b, inhibiting its ability to activate transcriptional elongation of the HIV viral genome (Yang et al., 2005). In human papilloma virus (HPV) infection, the binding of BRD4 CTD to HPV E2 protein acts to corepress HPV gene expression (Li, Guo, Wu, & Zhou, 2013; Zhu et al., 2012), a process required for latent infection. This same interaction between BRD4 and E2 protein, which allows BRD4 to tether E2 to the acetylated human chromatin, is exploited to facilitate equal segregation of viral episomes during mitosis.

Of the BET proteins, only BRD3 and BRD4 have been shown to play a direct role in human cancer pathogenesis. BRD3 and BRD4 drive NMC as oncoproteins (discussed in detail later), and BRD4 plays a significant role as a nononcogene in a large range of other cancers. Much of what is known of BRD4s involvement as an oncogene and nononcogene in cancer has been discovered through use of BET inhibitors as molecular probes, especially the JQ1 BET inhibitor created by Jay Bradner and his chemist, Jun Qi, for whom the molecule was named (Filippakopoulos et al., 2010). Since the introduction of JQ1, hundreds of papers have been published implicating a role of BRD4, including Burkitt and non-Burkitt lymphoma (Chapuy et al., 2013; Emadali et al., 2013; Mertz et al., 2011), acute leukemia (Zuber et al., 2011), multiple myeloma (Delmore et al., 2011), prostate cancer (Asangani et al., 2014), neuroblastoma (Puissant et al., 2013), medulloblastoma (Henssen et al., 2013), breast cancer (Crawford et al., 2008; Sengupta, Biarnes, Clarke, & Jordan, 2015), pancreatic cancer (Garcia et al., 2015; Mazur et al., 2015), ovarian cancer (Qiu et al., 2015), and nonsmall-cell carcinoma of the lung (Shimamura et al., 2013). BRD2 misexpression can eventually produce B-cell lymphoma in mice; however, there is no documentation of its involvement in human cancer (Greenwald et al., 2004).

3. BET INHIBITORS

Due to BRD4's broad role in cancer, inhibitors of the bromodomain of BET proteins have been developed with the purpose of therapeutically inhibiting BRD4-driven cancers. While these inhibitors affect all BET proteins, including BRDT, BRD2, BRD3, and BRD4, they have shown an unexpected degree of specificity for a variety of cancer pathways.

3.1 Discovery

The original BET inhibitors were thienodiazepine compounds developed by Yoshitomi Pharmaceuticals (now Mitsubishi Tanabe Pharma, Osaka, Japan) in the early 1990s in a screen to identify small molecules that could be used to treat autoimmune disease (Filippakopoulos et al., 2010). Bradner and colleagues, who were working with us to target BRD4–NUT pharmacologically, learned of the BET inhibitory properties of thienodiazepines and developed JQ1 to target BRD4–NUT, the fusion oncoprotein that drives NMC. The findings, which demonstrated the exquisite sensitivity of NMC cells to JQ1, formed the proof of principle that BET inhibitors indeed inhibit BRD4, and can potentially be used therapeutically, given their excellent pharmacologic properties (Filippakopoulos et al., 2010). At the same time of these studies, GlaxoSmithKline (GSK, Philadelphia, PA) developed their own BET inhibitors for a completely different purpose, and more in line with their original intent, to prevent septic shock (Nicodeme et al., 2010). Since then, GSK has come out with a BET inhibitor, iBET762, that is currently enrolling NMC and other cancer patients, and the Mitsubishi compound was purchased by OncoEthix (Lausanne, Switzerland, called OTX015, now owned by Merck, Kenilworth, NJ) and has been used to treat NMC and leukemia/lymphoma patients (Herait et al., 2014; Stathis et al., 2014). Since then, multiple pharmaceutical companies have developed BET inhibitors for cancer treatment with numerous ongoing clinical trials worldwide (Table 1). The results of those trials have yet-to-be published, however, the preliminary findings have been encouraging (Herait et al., 2014; Stathis et al., 2014).

3.2 Chemistry

BET inhibitors have a thienodiazepine backbone that is modified to not bind the central benzodiazepine receptor, and thus lack the psychotropic effects of benzodiazepines, but maintain their favorable pharmacologic properties. BET inhibitors are essentially acetyl-lysine mimetics that specifically bind the acetyl-lysine binding pocket of both bromodomains (Fig. 3, BD1 and BD2) of all BET proteins (BRDT, BRD2, BRD3, and BRD4), with high affinity (nM IC50); they have low affinity for bromodomains of non-BET proteins such as p300/CBP (Filippakopoulos et al., 2010; Nicodeme et al., 2010; Prinjha, Witherington, & Lee, 2012). Specific inhibitors that preferentially target one type of BET protein over others (eg, BRDT, but not BRD2–4) have not yet been identified.

Table 1 Clinical Trials Using BET Inhibitors in Cancer Clinical Trials.

gov Identifier	Cancer	Drug	Company	Phase	Start Date	Recruiting Locations
NCT02391480	Advanced cancer, breast cancer, nonsmall-cell lung cancer, acute myeloid leukemia, multiple myeloma	ABBV-075	AbbVie, Chicago, IL	1	Apr. 2015	Scottsdale, Arizona, United States; Indianapolis, Indiana, United States; Houston, Texas, United States
NCT02431260	Advanced cancer	INCB054329	Incyte Corporation, Alapocas, DE	1/2	May 2015	Los Angeles, California, United States; Denver, Colorado, United States; Chicago, Illinois, United States; Lafayette, Indiana, United States; Ann Arbor, Michigan, United States; Houston, Texas, United States
NCT02308761	Acute myeloid leukemia (AML), myelodysplastic syndrome (MDS)	TEN-010	Tensha Therapeutics, Cambridge, MA	1	Oct. 2014	Boston, Massachusetts, United States; New York, New York, United States
NCT01987362	NMC, advanced solid malignancies	TEN-010	Tensha Therapeutics	1	Oct. 2013	New Haven, Connecticut, United States; Boston, Massachusetts, United States; Detroit, Michigan, United States; Cleveland, Ohio, United States

NCT Number	Condition	Drug	Sponsor	Phase	Date	Locations
NCT02259114	NMC, triple negative breast cancer, nonsmall-cell lung cancer with rearranged ALK gene/fusion protein or KRAS mutation, castrate-resistant prostate cancer (CRPC), pancreatic ductal adenocarcinoma	OTX015/MK-8628	Oncoethix GmbH	1	Oct. 2014	Brussels, Belgium; Kirkland, Quebec, Canada; Paris, France; Madrid, Spain; Lucerne 6, Switzerland
NCT01949883	Lymphoma	CPI-0610	Constellation Pharmaceuticals, Cambridge, MA	1	Sep. 2013	Denver, Colorado, United States; Boston, Massachusetts, United States; Hackensack, New Jersey, United States; New York, New York, United States; Columbus, Ohio, United States; Nashville, Tennessee, United States
NCT02157636	Multiple myeloma	CPI-0610	Constellation Pharmaceuticals	1	Jul. 2014	Scottsdale, Arizona, United States; Boston, Massachusetts, United States; Philadelphia, Pennsylvania, United States; Nashville, Tennessee, United States
NCT02158858	Acute myelocytic leukemia, myelodysplastic syndrome (MDS), myelodysplastic/myeloproliferative neoplasm, unclassifiable myelofibrosis	CPI-0610	Constellation Pharmaceuticals	1	Jun. 2014	Lafayette, Indiana, United States; Boston, Massachusetts, United States; New York, New York, United States; Philadelphia, Pennsylvania, United States

Continued

Table 1 Clinical Trials Using BET Inhibitors in Cancer—cont'd
Clinical Trials.

gov Identifier	Cancer	Drug	Company	Phase	Start Date	Recruiting Locations
NCT02419417	Multiple indications cancer	BMS-986158	Bristol-Myers Squibb, Devens, MA	1/2a	Jun. 2015	Duarte, California, United States; Greenville, South Carolina, United States; Westmead, New South Wales, Australia; Melbourne, Victoria, Australia; Ottawa, Ontario, Canada
NCT02586155	Diabetes mellitus, type 2, coronary artery disease, cardiovascular diseases	RVX000222	Resverlogix Corp	3	Oct. 2015	Bonheiden, Belgium
NCT01587703	NMC, small-cell lung cancer (SCLC), nonsmall-cell lung cancer (NSCLC), colorectal cancer (CRC), neuroblastoma (NB), castration-resistant prostate cancer (CRPC), triple negative breast cancer (TNBC), estrogen receptor positive (ER positive) breast cancer	GSK525762	GlaxoSmithKline	1/2	Mar. 2012	Baltimore, Maryland, United States; Boston, Massachusetts, United States; Philadelphia, Pennsylvania, United States; Houston, Texas, United States; Bordeaux Cedex, France; Lyon Cedex 08, France; Barcelona, Spain; Madrid, Spain; Sutton, Surrey, United Kingdom; Newcastle upon Tyne, United Kingdom

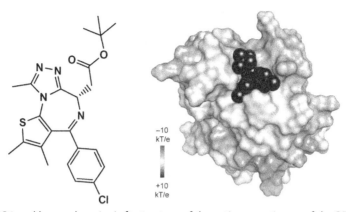

Fig. 3 JQ1 and bromodomain. *Left*, structure of the active enantiomer of the BET inhibitor, JQ1. *Right*, space filling model based on the high-resolution crystal structure of JQ1 (*yellow*) bound to bromodomain I of BRD4. *Adapted from Filippakopoulos, P., Qi, J., Picaud, S., Shen, Y., Smith, W. B., Fedorov, O., et al., (2010). Selective inhibition of BET bromodomains.* Nature, 468, 1067–1073. (See the color plate.)

3.3 Tolerability

A major concern for use of BET inhibitors as targeted therapy of cancer is that it is in theory a rather blunt, not precision instrument, inhibiting all BET proteins, some of which are required for fundamental cellular processes, and which are ubiquitously expressed throughout the body. The embryonic lethality of BRD2 and BRD4 homozygous knockouts in mice is evidence to support a lack of redundancy in the function of these proteins in development, further raising concerns in targeting these proteins clinically. In reality, the thienodiazepine BET inhibitors appear to be more tolerated than expected. Tumor-bearing mice given 50 mg/kg/day of JQ1 tolerate this regimen well for at least 30 days (Filippakopoulos et al., 2010). Humans with lymphoma or acute leukemia given 60 mg/day of the OncoEthix OTX015 BET inhibitor also tolerate the drug; however, thrombocytopenia is a common reversible toxicity (Stathis et al., 2014). It has been found that BRD3 binds to and activates the GATA-1 TF via bromodomain–acetyl-lysine interaction and that inhibition of this interaction by BET inhibitor can interfere with DNA targeting of GATA-1, resulting in transcriptional repression of erythroid and megakaryocytic gene transcription programs (Gamsjaeger et al., 2011; Lamonica et al., 2011). These findings may offer a possible mechanism for the thrombocytopenia seen in BET inhibitor-treated patients. Thus, the question remains whether a therapeutic window exists where drug levels sufficient to inhibit tumor growth are below dose-limiting toxicity. It is expected that results from ongoing clinical trials will be published soon, so that questions such as these will be answered.

Nevertheless, the toxicity of these BET inhibitors is less than would be expected for the inhibition of a general transcriptional regulator. A possible explanation is that BET inhibitors have nonuniform suppressive effects on transcription across the genome. While BRD4 is present at thousands of genomic sites, including the enhancers of all active genes (Anand et al., 2013; Loven et al., 2013; Zhang et al., 2012), JQ1 has only a modest effect on the transcription of the majority of these, but a marked effect on that of just a few hundred genes, including *MYC* and *BCL2*, in malignant hematologic cells (Anand et al., 2013; Dawson et al., 2011; Delmore et al., 2011; Devaiah et al., 2012; Loven et al., 2013; Mertz et al., 2011; Zuber et al., 2011). Moreover, the specific genes suppressed by BET inhibition is cell type dependent; MYC expression is inhibited in myeloma and other cancer cell types, but unaffected in fibroblasts (French et al., 2008; Zuber et al., 2011). The genes specifically sensitive to BET inhibition are typically associated with large clusters of enhancers highly enriched with Mediator, BRD4, and acetyl-histone H3K27 (H3K27Ac), and have been termed as super-enhancers (originally known as locus control regions) (Aronow et al., 1995; Caterina, Ciavatta, Donze, Behringer, & Townes, 1994; Loven et al., 2013). Super-enhancers, like enhancers, upregulate gene expression often through long-range interactions with the promoters of those genes (Herranz et al., 2014). Super-enhancers are thought to be cell lineage defining, and their targeting by BET inhibitors may explain the differential suppressive effects; however, the robustness and broad relevance of super-enhancer inhibition by BET inhibitors is a topic under active investigation (Adam et al., 2015; Shi & Vakoc, 2014).

The emergence of BET inhibitors has revealed the broad significance of super-enhancers in both disease-specific and developmental biology. Recent findings by Adam et al. (2015) using hair follicle development and wound healing as models have demonstrated that super-enhancers appear and disappear at different locations within the genome to enable changes in gene expression required for changes in cell phenotype that occur during these dynamic processes. The studies indicated that super-enhancers play a key role in the plasticity of expression of cell-type-specific genes required during development and healing (Adam et al., 2015). These findings demonstrate that not only are super-enhancers cell lineage defining but are also rapidly responsive to environmental and developmental signals, allowing for rapid changes in gene expression that coincide with changes in cell state. The key role of super-enhancers in cell dynamics raises the concern that BET inhibitors may impair adaptive cellular responses that require changes of cell state, such as those that occur during inflammation or wound healing. The known suppression of inflammation by BET inhibitors supports this possibility (Bandukwala et al., 2012; Mele et al., 2013; Nicodeme et al., 2010); however, the investigations have focused more on therapeutic effect on pathologic inflammation. It would be important to determine the deleterious effects, if any, of BET inhibitors on normal inflammation in response to infection, or wound healing.

4. BET INHIBITION IN NMC

As the only tumor to harbor an oncogene form of *BRD4* or *BRD3*, NMC is considered the prototype BET-driven cancer (Belkina & Denis, 2012; Chaidos et al., 2015; Shi & Vakoc, 2014). Thus, NMC is a logical disease to study both oncogenic BRD4 pathways, and the effects and mechanism of its inhibition. Much of the following will focus on mechanism of oncogenic BRD4 and BET inhibition in NMC.

4.1 NUT Midline Carcinoma

NMC is a rare subtype of squamous cell carcinoma defined by rearrangements of the *NUT*, aka *NUTM1*, gene on chromosome 15.q14. Most commonly the rearrangement is a translocation between *BRD4* (chr. 19p13.1) and *NUT*, forming the *BRD4–NUT*-fusion in 75–80% of cases (Bauer et al., 2012; French et al., 2003; Thompson-Wicking et al., 2013). NMC is one of the most aggressive solid tumor known, having a median survival of 6.7 months (Bauer et al., 2012). Uniquely for an aggressive carcinoma, NMC possesses simple cytogenetics, often with only a single translocation involving the *NUT* gene (French et al., 2003; Kees, Mulcahy, & Willoughby, 1991; Kubonishi et al., 1991; Lee et al., 1993). With no other known genetic aberrations, and its occurrence in children and neonates (French et al., 2004; Shehata et al., 2010), it is possible that the *NUT*-fusions act alone to drive growth of this cancer, representing a "genetic shortcut" to squamous cell carcinoma (French, 2012, 2014).

NMC most commonly arises in the thorax, and second most commonly and increasingly recognized in the head and neck. The name "midline" is based on the original observations that NMC arises from midline structures, including sinonasal (Stelow et al., 2008), pharyngeal (French et al., 2004), upper aerodigestive tract (Stelow et al., 2008), mediastinum/thymus

(Kubonishi et al., 1991), and even bladder (French et al., 2004). Multiple cases that have occurred outside the midline, including those involving bone (Mertens, Wiebe, Adlercreutz, Mandahl, & French, 2007), lung (Evans et al., 2012), pancreas (Shehata et al., 2010), and salivary glands (Davis et al., 2011), have challenged the notion of midline, and the World Health Organization classification of tumors has changed the name to NUT Carcinoma (French & den Bakker, 2015).

NMC was originally thought to be a disease of children and young adults (French et al., 2004), but is now well recognized to affect patients of all ages, including a range from neonates (Shehata et al., 2010) to patients in their eighth decade (French, 2012; Stelow et al., 2008).

The histology of NMC is that of a poorly differentiated malignant round cell neoplasm, often with the presence of focal squamous differentiation (French, 2012). This nonspecific histology can be confused with conventional squamous cell carcinoma, sinonasal undifferentiated carcinoma, Ewing sarcoma, small-cell carcinoma, and even acute leukemia (Evans et al., 2012; French, 2010, 2012; Mertens et al., 2007; Stelow et al., 2008). Thus, the diagnosis of NMC is not made based on histopathology alone. Fortunately, the definitive diagnostic test is an immunohistochemical (IHC) stain using a monoclonal antibody to NUT (clone C52, Cell Signaling Technologies, Danvers, MA) that can be used in any pathology laboratory (French & den Bakker, 2015). The diagnostic pattern is nuclear speckled staining of the majority of tumor cells, a phenomenon that actually has biological significance, as discussed later (Fig. 4A and B). As this stain is 100% specific and 87% sensitive (French & den Bakker, 2015; Haack et al., 2009) it is not necessary to confirm the diagnosis by other molecular means, such as those historically used including cytogenetics (Kees et al., 1991; Toretsky et al., 2003), reverse transcriptase PCR (Tanaka et al., 2012), fluorescent in situ hybridization (French et al., 2004), or next-generation sequencing (Stirnweiss et al., 2015). The reason for the high specificity of the NUT antibody is that wild-type NUT expression is exclusively restricted to postmeiotic spermatids and oocytes (French et al., 2003). In every case documented, the expression of NUT in NMC cells is driven not by the NUT promoter, but by its 5′ fusion partner (French et al., 2003; Stirnweiss et al., 2015; Thompson-Wicking et al., 2013), thus ectopic NUT expression is highly specific for NMC.

The value of performing molecular analysis is not in diagnosis or prognosis, but in the identification of the fusion partner to *NUT* as a research

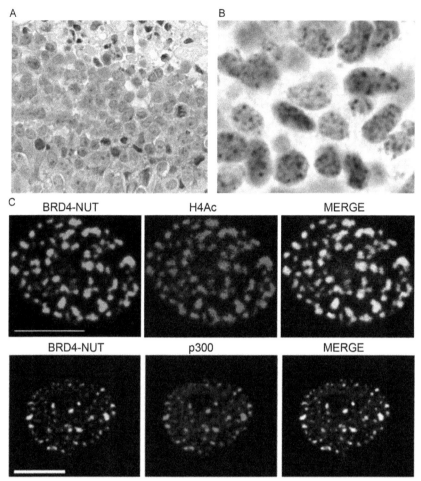

Fig. 4 BRD4–NUT foci colocalize with p300 and active chromatin. (A) Typical histologic appearance of an NMC reveals a high-grade carcinoma with necrosis and mitoses. (B) NUT immunohistochemistry reveals BRD4–NUT foci in a resected tumor. The findings are diagnostic of NMC. (C) Immunofluorescence from transgenically expressed BRD4–NUT reveals colocalization with p300 and acetyl-histones. *(C) Adapted from Reynoird, N., Schwartz, B. E., Delvecchio, M., Sadoul, K., Meyers, D., Mukherjee, C., et al. (2010). Oncogenesis by sequestration of CBP/p300 in transcriptionally inactive hyperacetylated chromatin domains. The EMBO Journal, 29, 2943–2952.* (See the color plate.)

inquiry. In fact, no study thus far has demonstrated a significantly different prognosis for the different *NUT*-fusion types (Bauer et al., 2012), though studies have been limited by low patient numbers and lack of statistical power. Apart from fusion to *BRD4*, *NUT* also can fuse to *BRD3*

(French et al., 2008) and *NSD3* (French et al., 2014; Kuroda et al., 2015; Suzuki et al., 2014) at a much lower frequency (Bauer et al., 2012; French et al., 2004). The existence of multiple *NUT*-fusion types raises the question of differential response to therapy; however, lack of systematic studies and low patient numbers have precluded this analysis. An obvious concern would be whether NSD3–NUT+ NMC tumors, lacking bromodomains, are sensitive to BET inhibitors. Fortunately, because NSD3 binds BRD4, and BRD4 is essential for NSD3–NUT oncogenic function (French et al., 2014), NSD3–NUT+ NMCs are predicted to be BET inhibitor sensitive. Indeed, the one tumor tested in vitro was sensitive to JQ1.

A major challenge for NMC is that because it is a newly described, rare disease that cannot easily be distinguished from other cancers and of which many pathologists and clinicians are unaware, it is vastly underdiagnosed. The markedly uneven geographic distribution of NMC cases is evidence of this fact (French, 2012). For example, to this author's knowledge, there have been more patients diagnosed with NMC who lived in Boston, Massachusetts than those combined from India, Russia, China, and the entire continent of Africa since this entity became known! To meet this challenge, a centralized international tumor registry, the NMC Registry (http://www.NMCRegistry.org) that collects patient demographic and outcome data and tissue was created in 2010 and has been a major source of clinical information and awareness for this disease (Bauer et al., 2012).

Because NMC is potentially treatable with BET inhibitors, it is important to know when to test for this diagnosis. For the pathologist, any noncutaneous poorly differentiated carcinoma, particularly one that possesses some squamous features, such as p63 or CK5 expression, should be tested by NUT IHC (French & den Bakker, 2015). For the clinician, for any distinctly rapidly growing and/or disseminating carcinoma, the pathologist should be made aware to rule out NMC.

Currently, the most effective treatment of NMC, for which the only cures have been seen, is complete resection if the disease is localized (Chau et al., 2014; Mertens et al., 2007). Even with the option of BET inhibitors, the recommendation is to initially and immediately treat by complete resection, when possible. This is usually only possible for head and neck tumors which present earlier. No chemotherapeutic or radiation therapy regimen has independently been shown to be effective (Bauer et al., 2012; Chau et al., 2014), thus there is much hope that BET inhibitors will be a more effective option, as discussed later.

4.2 BRD4–NUT Function

The presence of *NUT*-fusion genes is the hallmark of NMC. The best characterized and most common oncoprotein is BRD4–NUT. The knockdown of BRD3/4– and NSD3–NUT in patient-derived tumor cells leads to arrested growth and rapid squamous differentiation, indicating that the general function of NUT-fusions is to block differentiation and maintain growth (French et al., 2008, 2014). Included in all *BRD4*– and *BRD3*– *NUT*-fusions are the two bromodomains and ET domain of both BET-encoded fusion genes, and nearly the entire coding sequence of *NUT* (exons 2–7) (French et al., 2003, 2008; Haruki et al., 2005; Stirnweiss et al., 2015; Thompson-Wicking et al., 2013) (Fig. 1), indicating that each of these regions is indispensible for their oncogenic function.

Very little is known about NUT. It is a completely unstructured protein with two acidic putative transcriptional activation domains (AD), a nuclear localization, and nuclear export signal (French, 2012; French et al., 2008) (Fig. 1). CRM1-dependent nuclear-cytoplasmic shuttling of NUT is observed when it is transgenically expressed in either U2OS or 293 T cells (French et al., 2008). By contrast, BRD–NUT is exclusively nuclear because NUT is tethered to chromatin via BRD's bromodomains. The first AD of NUT has been shown to interact with the HAT, p300 (Reynoird et al., 2010). It has been hypothesized that the binding and activation of p300 HAT activity by NUT is a crucial early step in the replacement of histones with protamines in the process of chromatin compaction during spermiogenesis (French, 2012, 2014; Reynoird et al., 2010). Moreover, the NUT–p300 interaction is thought to be critical to the oncogenic function of BRD–NUT (Alekseyenko et al., 2015).

The tethering of NUT to acetylated chromatin by BRD3/4 bromodomains is required for its blockade of differentiation. Expression of the dual BRD4 bromodomains alone acts as a dominant negative to BRD4–NUT oncogenic function, inducing differentiation in patient NMC cells. Additionally, replacement of either or both of the acetyl-histone-binding asparagines with alanine (BD12 N140A and/or N433A) completely prevents the ability of the dual bromodomains from inducing differentiation (Grayson et al., 2014). The findings demonstrated that the acetyl-lysine–bromodomain interaction is crucial for the oncogenic function of BRD4–NUT. Thus, a model emerges of a HAT-recruiting module, NUT, tethered to chromatin by BRD4s bromodomains.

It was originally postulated that the BRD4–NUT–p300 complex may function in a feedforward manner through the recruitment of p300 to chromatin by BRD4–NUT, leading to further acetylation and recruitment of both factors, eventually forming massive regions of acetylated chromatin, BRD4–NUT, and p300. The end result would be to sequester p300 to progrowth genes, and away from genes that encode factors required for differentiation. In support of this idea, the nuclear foci seen in vivo NMC tumors correspond to foci of active histone hyperacetylation and p300 seen by immunofluorescence (Fig. 4C) (Reynoird et al., 2010; Yan, Diaz, Jiao, Wang, & You, 2011). Moreover, it was shown that expression of endogenous and transgenic BRD4–NUT is associated with global hypoacetylation and transcriptional repression, indicating that BRD4–NUT may have an overall repressive effect on transcription, possibly because BRD4–NUT sequesters p300 activity (Schwartz et al., 2011). Indeed, pharmacologic reversal of global histone hypoacetylation using HDAC inhibitors restored transcription of differentiation-specific genes and resulted in the differentiation and arrested growth of NMC cells in vitro and in vivo. As clinical proof of principle, a patient with disseminated NMC demonstrated arrested growth of his tumor when treated with single agent vorinostat, an HDAC inhibitor (Merck) (Schwartz et al., 2011). Since then, HDAC inhibitors (SAHA, aka Vorinostat, Merck) have been used in combination with chemotherapy for treatment of NMC, demonstrating some initial, but transient responses (Maher, Christensen, Yedururi, Bell, & Tarek, 2015 and unpublished observations).

Taking a closer look at the BRD4–NUT nuclear foci suspect of sequestering p300, we and collaborators performed chromatin immunoprecipitation next-generation sequencing (ChIP-seq) of BRD4–NUT transgenically expressed in naive 293 T cells and patient-derived NMC cells. We found that BRD4–NUT was highly enriched in massive contiguous regions of active acetylated chromatin (H3K9Ac, H3K14Ac, H3K27Ac, and H3K27Me3), extending 100 kilobases (kb) to 2 megabases (MB) in size (Alekseyenko et al., 2015). These regions likely correspond to the BRD4–NUT nuclear foci seen by IHC, and are termed "megadomains." By comparison, super-enhancers are on the scale of 10–20 kb, an order of 1–2 magnitudes smaller. These megadomains are also enriched with p300, consistent with the idea that p300 is sequestered by BRD4–NUT. In kinetic experiments studying the formation of megadomains in 293 T cells, megadomains were shown to often arise from enhancers, but interestingly, not super-enhancers (Alekseyenko et al., 2015). Spreading occurred rapidly over a 7-h period and was limited to CTCF-associated boundaries. These boundaries correspond to those of topologically associating domains (TADs), DNA regions conserved across species which allow for long-range looping and cross-talk among enhancers and genes within the TAD (Ciabrelli & Cavalli, 2015). TADs are considered critical for the coordinated expression of genomic regions during development. Recently, aberrations of TAD boundaries have been shown to cause developmental disorders, such as polydactyl (Lupianez et al., 2015). Thus, it has been proposed that full occupation of TADs by BRD4–NUT allows it to control entire gene regulatory regions that are critical to the growth of the tumor cell (Alekseyenko et al., 2015).

Two such megadomain-occupied TADs of particular interest in NMC were those associated with the *MYC* and *TP63* genes. In all four NMC cell lines tested, and additionally one corresponding patient tumor tissue, a megadomain was present within the *MYC* and *TP63* gene loci (Alekseyenko et al., 2015). Megadomains otherwise showed very little overlap among these NMCs. Both MYC and p63 have both been shown to be required for growth of NMC cell lines (Alekseyenko et al., 2015; Grayson et al., 2014). In fact MYC can in part replace the function of BRD4–NUT to prevent differentiation/arrested proliferation induced by the knockdown of BRD4–NUT (Grayson et al., 2014). The findings support a model wherein BRD4–NUT controls expression of target genes through complete occupation of their DNA regulatory regions in a feedforward process that involves recruitment of p300 to BRD4–NUT (Fig. 5). Indeed, de novo expression of BRD4–NUT in 293 T cells results in transcription of both coding and noncoding DNA within megadomains.

4.3 Inhibition of BRD4–NUT by BET Inhibitors

The earlier findings suggest that recruitment of HATs by BRD4–NUT may activate transcription in areas of megadomains and are compatible with the original model that this sequestration is done at the expense of transcription of regions outside megadomains. Nevertheless, all studies have focused on transcription within megadomains, not outside of them. A key tool in dissecting the relationship between BRD4–NUT megadomains and transcription is the BET inhibitor, JQ1. JQ1 evicts BRD4 and BRD4–NUT from chromatin within seconds to minutes (Filippakopoulos et al., 2010), and megadomains become depleted of BRD4–NUT within 4 h (Alekseyenko et al., 2015), allowing for the evaluation of direct consequences of BRD4–NUT inhibition. Alekseyenko et al. (2015) found that transcription was overall increased in megadomains relative to adjacent regions and that of

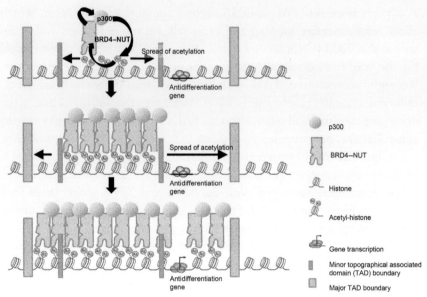

Fig. 5 Model of megadomain formation. *Adapted from Alekseyenko, A. A., Walsh, E. M., Wang, X., Grayson, A. R., Hsi, P. T., Kharchenko, P. V., et al. (2015). The oncogenic BRD4-NUT chromatin regulator drives aberrant transcription within large topological domains. Genes & Development, 29, 1507–1523.* (See the color plate.)

the majority of genes within megadomains decreased within 4 h of JQ1 treatment. *TP63* was one of the megadomain genes that decreased in transcription, but surprisingly *MYC* was not. Despite there being no effect on MYC RNA levels, MYC protein did decrease upon exposure to JQ1. A closer look at the *MYC* region revealed that several known *MYC* enhancers known to encode long noncoding RNAs (lncRNA), including multiple CCATs and PVT1 (Nagoshi et al., 2012; Tseng et al., 2014; Xiang et al., 2014), were transcriptionally active, and were exquisitely sensitive to JQ1. It is known that PVT1 lncRNA stabilizes MYC protein, and thus it was hypothesized that MYC expression is maintained at the protein level by BRD4–NUT through upregulation of PVT1. Indeed, PVT1 knockdown also led to decreased MYC protein and differentiation in NMC cells. The role of the other *MYC* enhancers and lncRNAs in the region upregulated by BRD4–NUT is not clear, but could also be posttranslational.

It is possible that there are other key gene targets of BRD4–NUT megadomains; however, ChIP-seq demonstrated that, apart from *MYC* and *TP63* loci, the majority of megadomain loci did not overlap between different

NMC cell lines. The findings suggest a "one shot" phenomenon where among many loci targeted, only a select few are relevant to the oncogenic function of BRD4–NUT.

4.4 Clinical Trials with BET Inhibitors

Given the dependence of BRD4–NUT function on its interaction with chromatin, it is not surprising that NMC cells are sensitive to BET inhibition. The effect of JQ1 on NMC cell growth in vitro is similar to that of BRD4–NUT knockdown: terminal differentiation, growth suppression, and apoptosis (Beesley et al., 2014; Filippakopoulos et al., 2010). In vivo, JQ1 administered at 50 mg/kg daily in three mouse xenograft models of NMC causes significant growth suppression and improved survival (Filippakopoulos et al., 2010). Excised tumors demonstrate differentiation as seen in vitro.

The on-target inhibition and in vitro and in vivo proof of biological activity of BET inhibitors provides a clear rationale for treatment of NMC with these compounds. Indeed, the first report describing treatment of NMC patients with BET inhibitor was recently published (Stathis et al., 2016). This work describes the outcomes of four NMC patients treated with OTX015 (60–80 mg, OncoEthix/Merck) on a compassionate basis, outside of a clinical trial. Overall the results demonstrated on-target activity of BET inhibitors in NMC and established the proof-of-principle that BRD4–NUT can be therapeutically targeted. Two of the patients had rapid tumor regression and symptomatic improvement, and a third patient's disease stabilized demonstrating metabolic response (Fig. 6). While all patients eventually progressed and died, two patients lived 18 and 19 months from the time of diagnosis, notably longer than the median survival of 6.7 months (Bauer et al., 2012). Moreover, one patient was one of only 2 of 31 NMC patients managed nonsurgically known to survive for more than 17 months (Bauer et al., 2012; Mertens et al., 2007). In two patients, post-treatment biopsies demonstrated squamous differentiation, consistent with the observation that BET inhibitors interfere with the blockade of differentiation sustained by BRD4–NUT (Filippakopoulos et al., 2010) (Fig. 6C and D). While the findings are encouraging, they do not yet establish that BET inhibitors can increase survival in NMC patients; however, they provide rationale for further clinical development of BET inhibitors in NMC.

The main toxicities were thrombocytopenia, seen in all patients, nausea, and fatigue. The thrombocytopenia was a significant problem in some

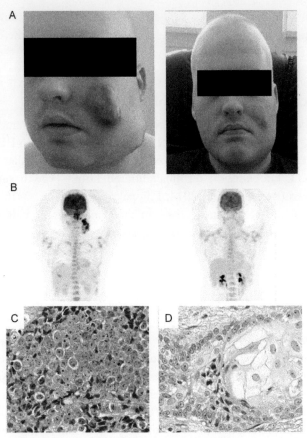

Fig. 6 Clinical benefit from treatment of 22-year-old NMC patient with OTX015 BET inhibitor. (A) *Left*, pre-BET inhibitor, and *right*, day 8 of the first cycle of treatment with OTX015/MK-8628. (B) PET at baseline (*left*) and PET after two cycles (*right*) shows disappearance of tumor uptake. (C) Pre-OTX015 biopsy of the patient's neck tumor reveals undifferentiated small-round *blue* cells. (D) Biopsy of the same lesion post-treatment reveals squamous differentiation demonstrated by stratification and accumulation of abundant cytoplasm, and pale nuclei, interpreted as prodifferentiative treatment effect. *Adapted from Stathis, A., Zucca, E., Bekradda, M., Gomez-Roca, C., Delord, J. P., de La Motte Rouge, T., et al. (2016). Clinical response of carcinomas harboring the BRD4-NUT oncoprotein to the targeted bromodomain inhibitor OTX015/MK-8628. Cancer Discovery (Epub ahead of print).* (See the color plate.)

patients, leading to treatment interruption and disease progression in one patient. On the whole, while BET inhibitors are effective, they may not be curative of NMC as single agent therapy, the main limitation being a narrow therapeutic window stemming from toxicity. Thus, combination approaches may be necessary as BET inhibitors are further developed.

Since the introduction of BET inhibitors in NMC, three phase I trials have emerged enrolling NMC patients, and multiple additional trials enrolling patients with hematologic and solid tumors (Table 1). The trials enrolling NMC patients include two in Europe treating patients with OTX015 and i–BET-762 (GSK) (Table 1). OTX015, there are three trials enrolling NMC patients in the United States for treatment with i–BET-762, Ten-10 (Tensha Therapeutics), and INCB054329 (Incyte Corporation). No results of these trials have been published yet, however, they are expected soon.

4.5 Other Cancers

The antineoplastic effects of BET inhibitors in NMC led to an explosion of investigations to determine the effects of BET inhibition in other cancers that do not harbor an oncogenic form of BRD4. It has been discovered that certain non–NMC cancers have a nononcogene addiction to nonmutated BRD4 for growth and viability. The dependency on BET proteins for growth and viability is predicted given the fundamental role these proteins serve in gene transcription. Surprisingly, however, the dependency is cell-type dependent, most likely because BET inhibitors have significant effects on only a small subset, $\sim$300, of cell-type-specific genes whose upregulation is maintained by super-enhancers (Loven et al., 2013). Fortunately, the cell-type specificity of BET inhibitors is such that the growth-dependent transcriptional programs that are inhibited by BET inhibitors in some cancer cell types are unaffected in other cell types, including some nonneoplastic cells (French et al., 2008; Zuber et al., 2011). The finding raises the possibility that BET inhibitors may be able to selectively target specific cancer cell types, while unaffecting nonneoplastic cells, however, this has not been extensively investigated and is an important issue that should be investigated in light of the emerging use of BET inhibitors.

BET inhibitors are effective at inhibiting MYC expression in multiple cancer types. MYC is one of the most common TFs implicated in driving cancer growth and since its discovery has been considered undruggable. In different cancers, MYC expression is controlled by cell-type-specific enhancers. In a prototypical example, the MM1.S multiple myeloma cell line, the *IgH* enhancer is fused to *MYC*, leading to its upregulation. The IgH enhancer in this line was found to be markedly enriched with BRD4, which is exquisitely sensitive to JQ1-induced depletion. JQ1 exposure leads to downregulation of MYC expression and inhibited proliferation in these cells (Delmore et al., 2011). Leukemia cells have their own *MYC* 3′ distal enhancers that are also markedly sensitive to JQ1, leading to downregulation of MYC expression (Dawson et al., 2011; Mertz et al., 2011; Zuber et al., 2011). The parallels with NMC, which have BET-inhibitor-sensitive MYC-associated megadomains, are obvious; however, in NMC it appears that multiple potential MYC enhancers are occupied by BRD4–NUT (Alekseyenko et al., 2015). One of these MYC enhancers, CCAT1, has been additionally implicated in colorectal carcinoma as a target of BET inhibitors that correlates with sensitivity to JQ1 (McCleland et al., 2016). Over the past 5 years, it has become evident that the sensitivity of a wide range of cancers to BET inhibition is due to targeting of MYC. Included in the growing list are non-Hodgkin and Burkitt lymphoma (Emadali et al., 2013; Mertz et al., 2011), medulloblastoma (Henssen et al., 2013), ovarian cancer (Qiu et al., 2015), hepatocellular carcinoma (Li et al., 2015), and possibly pancreatic cancer (Mazur et al., 2015).

The growth of castration-resistant prostate cancer (CRPC) is also inhibited by BET inhibitors. In CRPC, however, the growth inhibition by BET inhibitors is only in part due to effects on MYC expression. Asangani et al. (2014) found that JQ1 inhibits the interaction between BRD2/3/4 and the androgen receptor (AR), preventing the recruitment of AR to target genes, such as TMPRSS2-ERG. The effects of multitarget inhibition of CRPC cells by JQ1 became evident in vivo in xenografted tumors, where JQ1 treatment was more potent than AR antagonists.

BET inhibition of some lung cancers also appears independent of MYC. In a subset of lung adenocarcinomas that were exceptionally sensitive to JQ1, treatment correlated with downregulation of FOSL1 and its targets (Lockwood, Zejnullahu, Bradner, & Varmus, 2012), and not MYC. Likewise, *MYCN*-amplified neuroblastoma are inhibited through downregulation of MYCN and not MYC (Puissant et al., 2013).

Based on the compelling studies earlier, trials enrolling patients with a wide range of blood and solid tumors for treatment with BET inhibitors are ongoing (Table 1). Thus far, the results of one ongoing trial have been published in abstract form and are encouraging. In this trial enrolling patients with hematologic malignancies for treatment with OTX015, among 28 patients who were evaluable for response, two patients with acute myelogenous leukemia (AML) demonstrated a complete remission, and two patients with lymphoma had a partial remission (Herait et al., 2014). The most serious toxicity seen was reversible grade 3–4 thrombocytopenia in three patients.

5. RESISTANCE TO BET INHIBITORS

Resistance to small-molecule inhibitor cancer therapy is an inevitable complication of most targeted approaches and BET inhibitors are unlikely to be an exception. Indeed, models of resistance to BET inhibitors have already been reported, and the mechanisms of resistance differ for different cancer types. Recently, two groups revealed a novel mechanism for leukemic resistance to BET inhibitors (Fong et al., 2015; Rathert et al., 2015). The studies independently determined that the antiproliferative effects of BET inhibition can be overcome by activation of the Wnt/β-catenin pathway. Fong et al. (2015), using an RNAi screen, demonstrated that downregulation of the polycomb repressive complex 2 (PRC2), specifically Suz12, leads to derepression of Wnt/β-catenin signaling which upregulates MYC expression through compensatory activation of the *PVT1* enhancer of *MYC*. Importantly, the resistance to BET inhibition occurred despite continued inhibition of BRD4 targets, thus BRD4-dependence is bypassed. Parenthetically, the earlier mechanism overlaps that of BRD4–NUT megadomains, which also activate the *PVT1* enhancer (Alekseyenko et al., 2015, earlier).

Triple negative breast cancer (TNBC) was recently shown by Shu et al. (2016) to utilize a completely different mechanism of resistance to BET inhibition. In resistant TNBC, unlike resistant leukemia, the tumor cells remained completely dependent upon BRD4, which was bound to the same promoters and enhancers as the parental, BET-inhibitor-sensitive cell line. In this unique mechanism, BRD4 overcame BET inhibition through constitutive phosphorylation, causing it to bind with greater affinity to MED1, and thereby engage in the same genomic targets through "piggybacking" on the Mediator complex. The authors described the mechanism of constitutive phosphorylation to be through downregulation of the PP2A tumor suppressor phosphatase.

Would it be possible for BRD4–NUT to be resistant to BET inhibition in NMC, which is thought to be entirely dependent on this oncoprotein? In unpublished work, we have attempted to develop resistance to JQ1 in two cultured NMC cell lines using established methods for up to 9 months (Engelman et al., 2007) and have not succeeded. The findings may suggest that it is not possible for NMC to acquire resistance to BET inhibitors, and even further support a compelling rationale for targeting NMC with BET inhibitors. However, there is extensive evidence, based on in vitro IC50 values, that NMCs may not be any more sensitive to BET inhibitors than some BET-inhibitor-sensitive non-NMC tumors (Beesley et al., 2014; Filippakopoulos et al., 2010; Zuber et al., 2011). A possible cause for less-than-expected sensitivity of NMC to BET inhibition may lie in the structure of megadomains, which are massive, hyperacetylated regions that may have higher affinity to BRD4–NUT than super-enhancers. Recall that BRD4 binds with greater affinity to densely acetylated histones. Indeed, fluorescence recovery after photobleaching studies we performed indicated that the mobility of BRD4 on chromatin is twofold that of BRD4–NUT, suggesting a higher affinity interaction of BRD4–NUT with megadomains (French et al., 2008). The findings may explain the narrow therapeutic window for BET inhibitor treatment of NMC patients (Stathis et al., 2016).

6. FUTURE OF BET INHIBITORS

Based on the strong scientific rationale, preclinical, and clinical studies, there is hope that BET inhibitors will be effective at treating a subset of cancers. As with most drugs, it is likely therapy can be optimized using either next-generation BET inhibitors or through combinatorial strategies. This section will delve into a few of the most recent developments combining BET inhibitors with other compounds and new BET inhibitor derivatives.

6.1 Combinations

Given that BRD4-dependent transcriptional elongation requires the reading of chromatin by BRD4, investigators have reasoned that BRD4 dependency can be enhanced by hyperacetylating histones artificially, with the use of HDAC inhibitors (Fiskus, Sharma, Qi, Valenta, et al., 2014). Whether or not this is the mechanism, HDAC inhibitors have been found to synergize with BET inhibitors to inhibit growth and induce apoptosis in a number of in vitro and in vivo cancer models, including *MYCN*-amplified neuroblastoma (Shahbazi et al., 2016), pancreatic ductal adenocarcinoma (Mazur et al., 2015), invasive ductal carcinoma of the breast (Borbely, Haldosen, Dahlman-Wright, & Zhao, 2015), melanoma (Heinemann et al., 2015), and AML (Fiskus, Sharma, Qi, Valenta, et al., 2014).

Along the same lines of targeting BRD4-dependent transcriptional elongation, investigators have focused on the so-called super-enhancer complex (SEC) of which BRD4 plays a pivotal role. The SEC includes BRD4, HDACs, HMT, and P-TEFb (CDK9/cyclin T1), which together are required for transcriptional programs that drive tumor growth. As described earlier (Section 2.2 BET Function, Fig. 2), transcriptional elongation is dependent upon recruitment of P-TEFb by BRD4. Thus, Bahr and Colleagues (2015) tested whether combinations of a BET inhibitor (JQ1) and CDK9 inhibitor (Alvocidib, Tolero Pharmaceuticals) would synergize to inhibit BRD4 function and tumorigenesis. Indeed potent BRD4 inhibition was seen through complete elimination of MYC RNA expression, and the two compounds synergized to inhibit tumor growth in both an in vitro and in vivo model of AML.

In another context, BET inhibitors have been used to overcome kinase inhibitor resistance in several cancer models. Studies have shown that BET inhibitors blunt adaptive kinome responses to kinase inhibitors, thus abrogating resistance. Specifically, resistance has been overcome in Her2/neu + lapatinib-resistant breast cancer cells combining lapatinib (Her2/neu and EGFR tyrosine kinase inhibitor) and BET inhibitor (Stuhlmiller et al., 2015). The combination of ponatinib or AC220 (FLT3 tyrosine kinase inhibitors) with JQ1 has overcome FLT3-resistant AML (Fiskus, Sharma, Qi, Shah, et al., 2014); and GDC-0941 (PI3 kinase inhibitor) combined with JQ1 has overcome PI3 kinase inhibitor resistance in breast cancer cells (Stratikopoulos et al., 2015).

6.2 Novel BET Inhibitor Derivatives

Just as combination therapeutic approaches are emerging, so are novel strategies to improve the molecular design of BET inhibitors. One such breakthrough recently was made by Winter et al. (2015). This group built on the recent discovery that explains the mechanism of inhibition of phthalimide drugs (such as thalidomide) in multiple myeloma. Lu et al. (2014) had shown that the cereblon (CRBN) component of a cullin–RING ubiquitin E3 ligase complex binds thalidomide, creating an interface that recruits B-cell-specific Ikaros TFs (Fischer et al., 2014) for proteosomal degradation. Winter et al. took advantage of this property of thalidomide to target BET proteins for CRBN-dependent proteosomal degradation by creating a bifunctional JQ1 molecule fused to thalidomide, termed dBET. dBET specifically targeted BET proteins for destruction, leading to higher levels of apoptosis of primary AML cells than those treated with JQ1 alone. Inhibition was also seen in vivo in mice xenografts (Lu et al., 2014). The dBET type molecules may potentially be more effective than current BET inhibitors at preventing resistance, because at least some BET-inhibitor-resistant cancers (perhaps not leukemia) remain dependent on BRD4 (Shu et al., 2016).

7. CONCLUDING REMARKS

BET inhibitors are one of an emerging group of small-molecule inhibitors targeting transcription complex components. They arise as powerful tools to probe epigenetic mechanisms in cancer and are tolerated well enough to be used therapeutically as antineoplastic agents. Clinical studies have revealed some encouraging results in blood cancers; however, it is too early to determine whether current BET inhibitors are effective cancer therapies. It is likely that toxicity and resistance will occur, and studies are underway testing synergistic combinations with BET inhibitors to increase potency and overcome resistance. Moreover, novel BET inhibitor derivatives show promise to circumvent resistance in cancers that remain BRD4 dependent.

REFERENCES

Adam, R. C., Yang, H., Rockowitz, S., Larsen, S. B., Nikolova, M., Oristian, D. S., et al. (2015). Pioneer factors govern super-enhancer dynamics in stem cell plasticity and lineage choice. *Nature, 521,* 366–370.

Alekseyenko, A. A., Walsh, E. M., Wang, X., Grayson, A. R., Hsi, P. T., Kharchenko, P. V., et al. (2015). The oncogenic BRD4-NUT chromatin regulator drives aberrant transcription within large topological domains. *Genes & Development, 29,* 1507–1523.

Anand, P., Brown, J. D., Lin, C. Y., Qi, J., Zhang, R., Artero, P. C., et al. (2013). BET bromodomains mediate transcriptional pause release in heart failure. *Cell, 154,* 569–582.

Aronow, B. J., Ebert, C. A., Valerius, M. T., Potter, S. S., Wiginton, D. A., Witte, D. P., et al. (1995). Dissecting a locus control region: Facilitation of enhancer function by extended enhancer-flanking sequences. *Molecular Cell. Biology, 15,* 1123–1135.

Asangani, I. A., Dommeti, V. L., Wang, X., Malik, R., Cieslik, M., Yang, R., et al. (2014). Therapeutic targeting of BET bromodomain proteins in castration-resistant prostate cancer. *Nature, 510,* 278–282.

Bahr, B. L., Maughan, K. S., Soh, K. K., Bearss, J. J., Kim, W., Peterson, P., et al. (2015 Apr 18–22). Combination strategies to target super enhancer transcriptional activity by CDK9 and BRD4 inhibition in acute myeloid leukemia. In *Proceedings of the 106th Annual Meeting of the American Association for Cancer Research, Philadelphia, PA. Philadelphia (PA): AACR Cancer Research. 75* (15 Suppl.), 2015, Abstract number 2698.

Bandukwala, H. S., Gagnon, J., Togher, S., Greenbaum, J. A., Lamperti, E. D., Parr, N. J., et al. (2012). Selective inhibition of CD4 + T-cell cytokine production and autoimmunity by BET protein and c-Myc inhibitors. *Proceedings of the National Academy of Sciences of the United States of America, 109,* 14532–14537.

Bauer, D., Mitchell, C., Strait, K., Lathan, C., Stelow, E., Lueer, S., et al. (2012). Clinico-pathologic features and long-term outcomes of nut midline carcinoma. *Clinical Cancer Research, 18,* 5773–5779.

Beesley, A. H., Stirnweiss, A., Ferrari, E., Endersby, R., Howlett, M., Failes, T. W., et al. (2014). Comparative drug screening in NUT midline carcinoma. *British Journal of Cancer, 110,* 1189–1198.

Belkina, A. C., & Denis, G. V. (2012). BET domain co-regulators in obesity, inflammation and cancer. *Nature Reviews Cancer, 12,* 465–477.

Belkina, A. C., Nikolajczyk, B. S., & Denis, G. V. (2013). BET protein function is required for inflammation: Brd2 genetic disruption and BET inhibitor JQ1 impair mouse macrophage inflammatory responses. *The Journal of Immunology, 190,* 3670–3678.

Bisgrove, D. A., Mahmoudi, T., Henklein, P., & Verdin, E. (2007). Conserved P-TEFb-interacting domain of BRD4 inhibits HIV transcription. *Proceedings of the National Academy of Sciences of the United States of America, 104,* 13690–13695.

Borbely, G., Haldosen, L. A., Dahlman-Wright, K., & Zhao, C. (2015). Induction of USP17 by combining BET and HDAC inhibitors in breast cancer cells. *Oncotarget, 6,* 33623–33635.

Caterina, J. J., Ciavatta, D. J., Donze, D., Behringer, R. R., & Townes, T. M. (1994). Multiple elements in human beta-globin locus control region 5' HS 2 are involved in enhancer activity and position-independent, transgene expression. *Nucleic Acids Research, 22,* 1006–1011.

Chaidos, A., Caputo, V., & Karadimitris, A. (2015). Inhibition of bromodomain and extraterminal proteins (BET) as a potential therapeutic approach in haematological malignancies: Emerging preclinical and clinical evidence. *Therapeutic Advances in Hematology, 6,* 128–141.

Chapuy, B., McKeown, M. R., Lin, C. Y., Monti, S., Roemer, M. G., Qi, J., et al. (2013). Discovery and characterization of super-enhancer-associated dependencies in diffuse large B cell lymphoma. *Cancer Cell, 24,* 777–790.

Chase, A., & Cross, N. C. (2011). Aberrations of EZH2 in cancer. *Clinical Cancer Research, 17,* 2613–2618.

Chau, N. G., Mitchell, C. M., Aserlind, A., Grunfeld, N., Kaplan, L., Bauer, D. E., et al. (2014). Aggressive treatment and survival outcomes in NUT midline carcinoma (NMC) of the head and neck (HN). *Journal of Clinical Oncology, 32.* 2014 ASCO Annual Meeting Abstracts.

Ciabrelli, F., & Cavalli, G. (2015). Chromatin-driven behavior of topologically associating domains. *Journal of Molecular Biology, 427,* 608–625.

Crawford, N. P., Alsarraj, J., Lukes, L., Walker, R. C., Officewala, J. S., Yang, H. H., et al. (2008). Bromodomain 4 activation predicts breast cancer survival. *Proceedings of the National Academy of Sciences of the United States of America, 105,* 6380–6385.

Crowley, T. E., Kaine, E. M., Yoshida, M., Nandi, A., & Wolgemuth, D. J. (2002). Reproductive cycle regulation of nuclear import, euchromatic localization, and association with components of Pol II mediator of a mammalian double-bromodomain protein. *Molecular Endocrinology, 16,* 1727–1737.

Dash, A., & Gilliland, D. G. (2001). Molecular genetics of acute myeloid leukaemia. *Best Practice & Research Clinical Haematology, 14,* 49–64.

Davis, B. N., Karabakhtsian, R. G., Pettigrew, A. L., Arnold, S. M., French, C. A., & Brill, Y. M. (2011). Nuclear protein in testis midline carcinomas: A lethal and under-recognized entity. *Archives of Pathology & Laboratory Medicine, 135,* 1494–1498.

Dawson, M. A., Prinjha, R. K., Dittmann, A., Giotopoulos, G., Bantscheff, M., Chan, W. I., et al. (2011). Inhibition of BET recruitment to chromatin as an effective treatment for MLL-fusion leukaemia. *Nature, 478,* 529–533.

Deb, G., Thakur, V. S., & Gupta, S. (2013). Multifaceted role of EZH2 in breast and prostate tumorigenesis: Epigenetics and beyond. *Epigenetics, 8,* 464–476.

Delmore, J. E., Issa, G. C., Lemieux, M. E., Rahl, P. B., Shi, J., Jacobs, H. M., et al. (2011). BET bromodomain inhibition as a therapeutic strategy to target c-Myc. *Cell, 146,* 904–917.

Denis, G. V. (2010). Bromodomain coactivators in cancer, obesity, type 2 diabetes, and inflammation. *Discovery Medicine, 10,* 489–499.

Denis, G. V., & Green, M. R. (1996). A novel, mitogen-activated nuclear kinase is related to a Drosophila developmental regulator. *Genes & Development, 10*, 261–271.

Denis, G. V., McComb, M. E., Faller, D. V., Sinha, A., Romesser, P. B., & Costello, C. E. (2006). Identification of transcription complexes that contain the double bromodomain protein Brd2 and chromatin remodeling machines. *Journal of Proteome Research, 5*, 502–511.

Denis, G. V., Vaziri, C., Guo, N., & Faller, D. V. (2000). RING3 kinase transactivates promoters of cell cycle regulatory genes through E2F. *Cell Growth & Differentiation, 11*, 417–424.

Devaiah, B. N., Lewis, B. A., Cherman, N., Hewitt, M. C., Albrecht, B. K., Robey, P. G., et al. (2012). BRD4 is an atypical kinase that phosphorylates serine2 of the RNA polymerase II carboxy-terminal domain. *Proceedings of the National Academy of Sciences of the United States of America, 109*, 6927–6932.

Dey, A., Chitsaz, F., Abbasi, A., Misteli, T., & Ozato, K. (2003). The double bromodomain protein Brd4 binds to acetylated chromatin during interphase and mitosis. *Proceedings of the National Academy of Sciences of the United States of America, 100*, 8758–8763.

Dey, A., Ellenberg, J., Farina, A., Coleman, A. E., Maruyama, T., Sciortino, S., et al. (2000). A bromodomain protein, MCAP, associates with mitotic chromosomes and affects G(2)-to-M transition. *Molecular Cell. Biology, 20*, 6537–6549.

Dey, A., Nishiyama, A., Karpova, T., McNally, J., & Ozato, K. (2009). Brd4 marks select genes on mitotic chromatin and directs postmitotic transcription. *Molecular Biology of the Cell, 20*, 4899–4909.

Dhalluin, C., Carlson, J. E., Zeng, L., He, C., Aggarwal, A. K., & Zhou, M. M. (1999). Structure and ligand of a histone acetyltransferase bromodomain. *Nature, 399*, 491–496.

Digan, M. E., Haynes, S. R., Mozer, B. A., Dawid, I. B., Forquignon, F., & Gans, M. (1986). Genetic and molecular analysis of fs(1)h, a maternal effect homeotic gene in Drosophila. *Developmental Biology, 114*, 161–169.

Emadali, A., Rousseaux, S., Bruder-Costa, J., Rome, C., Duley, S., Hamaidia, S., et al. (2013). Identification of a novel BET bromodomain inhibitor-sensitive, gene regulatory circuit that controls Rituximab response and tumour growth in aggressive lymphoid cancers. *EMBO Molecular Medicine, 5*, 1180–1195.

Engelman, J. A., Zejnullahu, K., Mitsudomi, T., Song, Y., Hyland, C., Park, J. O., et al. (2007). MET amplification leads to gefitinib resistance in lung cancer by activating ERBB3 signaling. *Science, 316*, 1039–1043.

Evans, A. G., French, C. A., Cameron, M. J., Fletcher, C. D., Jackman, D. M., Lathan, C. S., et al. (2012). Pathologic characteristics of nut midline carcinoma arising in the mediastinum. *The American Journal of Surgical Pathology, 36*, 1222–1227.

Filippakopoulos, P., & Knapp, S. (2012). The bromodomain interaction module. *FEBS Letters, 586*, 2692–2704.

Filippakopoulos, P., Picaud, S., Mangos, M., Keates, T., Lambert, J. P., Barsyte-Lovejoy, D., et al. (2012). Histone recognition and large-scale structural analysis of the human bromodomain family. *Cell, 149*, 214–231.

Filippakopoulos, P., Qi, J., Picaud, S., Shen, Y., Smith, W. B., Fedorov, O., et al. (2010). Selective inhibition of BET bromodomains. *Nature, 468*, 1067–1073.

Fischer, E. S., Bohm, K., Lydeard, J. R., Yang, H., Stadler, M. B., Cavadini, S., et al. (2014). Structure of the DDB1-CRBN E3 ubiquitin ligase in complex with thalidomide. *Nature, 512*, 49–53.

Fiskus, W., Sharma, S., Qi, J., Shah, B., Devaraj, S. G., Leveque, C., et al. (2014a). BET protein antagonist JQ1 is synergistically lethal with FLT3 tyrosine kinase inhibitor (TKI) and overcomes resistance to FLT3-TKI in AML cells expressing FLT-ITD. *Molecular Cancer Therapeutics, 13*, 2315–2327.

Fiskus, W., Sharma, S., Qi, J., Valenta, J. A., Schaub, L. J., Shah, B., et al. (2014b). Highly active combination of BRD4 antagonist and histone deacetylase inhibitor against human acute myelogenous leukemia cells. *Molecular Cancer Therapeutics, 13*, 1142–1154.

Floyd, S. R., Pacold, M. E., Huang, Q., Clarke, S. M., Lam, F. C., Cannell, I. G., et al. (2013). The bromodomain protein Brd4 insulates chromatin from DNA damage signalling. *Nature, 498*, 246–250.

Fong, C. Y., Gilan, O., Lam, E. Y., Rubin, A. F., Ftouni, S., Tyler, D., et al. (2015). BET inhibitor resistance emerges from leukaemia stem cells. *Nature, 525*, 538–542.

French, C. A. (2010). Demystified molecular pathology of NUT midline carcinomas. *Journal of Clinical Pathology, 63*, 492–496.

French, C. A. (2012). Pathogenesis of NUT midline carcinoma. *Annual Review of Pathology, 7*, 247–265.

French, C. (2014). NUT midline carcinoma. *Nature Reviews Cancer, 14*, 149–150.

French, C. A., & den Bakker, M. A. (2015). *NUT carcinoma.* Lyon, France: International Agency for Research on Cancer (IARC).

French, C. A., Kutok, J. L., Faquin, W. C., Toretsky, J. A., Antonescu, C. R., Griffin, C. A., et al. (2004). Midline carcinoma of children and young adults with NUT rearrangement. *Journal of Clinical Oncology, 22*, 4135–4139.

French, C. A., Miyoshi, I., Aster, J. C., Kubonishi, I., Kroll, T. G., Dal Cin, P., et al. (2001). BRD4 bromodomain gene rearrangement in aggressive carcinoma with translocation t (15;19). *The American Journal of Pathology, 159*, 1987–1992.

French, C. A., Miyoshi, I., Kubonishi, I., Grier, H. E., Perez-Atayde, A. R., & Fletcher, J. A. (2003). BRD4-NUT fusion oncogene: A novel mechanism in aggressive carcinoma. *Cancer Research, 63*, 304–307.

French, C. A., Rahman, S., Walsh, E. M., Kuhnle, S., Grayson, A. R., Lemieux, M. E., et al. (2014). NSD3-NUT fusion oncoprotein in NUT midline carcinoma: Implications for a novel oncogenic mechanism. *Cancer Discovery, 4*, 928–941.

French, C. A., Ramirez, C. L., Kolmakova, J., Hickman, T. T., Cameron, M. J., Thyne, M. E., et al. (2008). BRD-NUT oncoproteins: A family of closely related nuclear proteins that block epithelial differentiation and maintain the growth of carcinoma cells. *Oncogene, 27*, 2237–2242.

Gamsjaeger, R., Webb, S. R., Lamonica, J. M., Billin, A., Blobel, G. A., & Mackay, J. P. (2011). Structural basis and specificity of acetylated transcription factor GATA1 recognition by BET family bromodomain protein Brd3. *Molecular Cell. Biology, 31*, 2632–2640.

Garcia, P. L., Miller, A. L., Kreitzburg, K. M., Council, L. N., Gamblin, T. L., Christein, J. D., et al. (2015). The BET bromodomain inhibitor JQ1 suppresses growth of pancreatic ductal adenocarcinoma in patient-derived xenograft models. *Oncogene, 35*, 833–845.

Grayson, A. R., Walsh, E. M., Cameron, M. J., Godec, J., Ashworth, T., Ambrose, J. M., et al. (2014). MYC, a downstream target of BRD-NUT, is necessary and sufficient for the blockade of differentiation in NUT midline carcinoma. *Oncogene, 33*, 1736–1742.

Greenwald, R. J., Tumang, J. R., Sinha, A., Currier, N., Cardiff, R. D., Rothstein, T. L., et al. (2004). E mu-BRD2 transgenic mice develop B-cell lymphoma and leukemia. *Blood, 103*, 1475–1484.

Gyuris, A., Donovan, D. J., Seymour, K. A., Lovasco, L. A., Smilowitz, N. R., Halperin, A. L., et al. (2009). The chromatin-targeting protein Brd2 is required for neural tube closure and embryogenesis. *Biochimica et Biophysica Acta, 1789*, 413–421.

Haack, H., Johnson, L. A., Fry, C. J., Crosby, K., Polakiewicz, R. D., Stelow, E. B., et al. (2009). Diagnosis of NUT midline carcinoma using a NUT-specific monoclonal antibody. *The American Journal of Surgical Pathology, 33*, 984–991.

Hargreaves, D. C., Horng, T., & Medzhitov, R. (2009). Control of inducible gene expression by signal-dependent transcriptional elongation. *Cell, 138*, 129–145.

Haruki, N., Kawaguchi, K. S., Eichenberger, S., Massion, P. P., Gonzalez, A., Gazdar, A. F., et al. (2005). Cloned fusion product from a rare t(15;19)(q13.2;p13.1) inhibit S phase in vitro. *Journal of Medical Genetics, 42*, 558–564.

Heinemann, A., Cullinane, C., De Paoli-Iseppi, R., Wilmott, J. S., Gunatilake, D., Madore, J., et al. (2015). Combining BET and HDAC inhibitors synergistically induces apoptosis of melanoma and suppresses AKT and YAP signaling. *Oncotarget, 6,* 21507–21521.

Henssen, A., Thor, T., Odersky, A., Heukamp, L., El-Hindy, N., Beckers, A., et al. (2013). BET bromodomain protein inhibition is a therapeutic option for medulloblastoma. *Oncotarget, 4,* 2080–2095.

Herait, P. E., Berthon, C., Thieblemont, C., et al. (2014 Apr 5–9). Abstract CT231: BETbromodomain inhibitor OTX015 shows clinically meaningful activity at nontoxic doses: Interim results of an ongoing phase I trial in hematologic malignancies. In *Proceedings of the 105th Annual Meeting of the American Association for Cancer Research, San Diego, CA. Philadelphia (PA): AACR Cancer Research. 74* (19 Suppl.), 2014, Abstract number CT231.

Herranz, D., Ambesi-Impiombato, A., Palomero, T., Schnell, S. A., Belver, L., Wendorff, A. A., et al. (2014). A NOTCH1-driven MYC enhancer promotes T cell development, transformation and acute lymphoblastic leukemia. *Nature Medicine, 20,* 1130–1137.

Houzelstein, D., Bullock, S. L., Lynch, D. E., Grigorieva, E. F., Wilson, V. A., & Beddington, R. S. (2002). Growth and early postimplantation defects in mice deficient for the bromodomain-containing protein Brd4. *Molecular Cell. Biology, 22,* 3794–3802.

Jang, M. K., Mochizuki, K., Zhou, M., Jeong, H. S., Brady, J. N., & Ozato, K. (2005). The bromodomain protein Brd4 is a positive regulatory component of P-TEFb and stimulates RNA polymerase II-dependent transcription. *Molecular Cell, 19,* 523–534.

Jiang, Y. W., Veschambre, P., Erdjument-Bromage, H., Tempst, P., Conaway, J. W., Conaway, R. C., et al. (1998). Mammalian mediator of transcriptional regulation and its possible role as an end-point of signal transduction pathways. *Proceedings of the National Academy of Sciences of the United States of America, 95,* 8538–8543.

Kanno, T., Kanno, Y., Siegel, R. M., Jang, M. K., Lenardo, M. J., & Ozato, K. (2004). Selective recognition of acetylated histones by bromodomain proteins visualized in living cells. *Molecular Cell, 13,* 33–43.

Kees, U. R., Mulcahy, M. T., & Willoughby, M. L. (1991). Intrathoracic carcinoma in an 11-year-old girl showing a translocation t(15;19). *The American Journal of Pediatric Hematology/Oncology, 13,* 459–464.

Kubonishi, I., Takehara, N., Iwata, J., Sonobe, H., Ohtsuki, Y., Abe, T., et al. (1991). Novel t(15;19)(q15;p13) chromosome abnormality in a thymic carcinoma. *Cancer Research, 51,* 3327–3328.

Kuroda, S., Suzuki, S., Kurita, A., Muraki, M., Aoshima, Y., Tanioka, F., et al. (2015). Cytological features of a variant NUT midline carcinoma of the lung harboring the NSD3-NUT fusion gene: A case report and literature review. *Case Reports in Pathology, 2015.* 572951.

Kwak, H., & Lis, J. T. (2013). Control of transcriptional elongation. *Annual Review of Genetics, 47,* 483–508.

Lamonica, J. M., Deng, W., Kadauke, S., Campbell, A. E., Gamsjaeger, R., Wang, H., et al. (2011). Bromodomain protein Brd3 associates with acetylated GATA1 to promote its chromatin occupancy at erythroid target genes. *Proceedings of the National Academy of Sciences of the United States of America, 108,* E159–E168.

Lee, A. C., Kwong, Y. I., Fu, K. H., Chan, G. C., Ma, L., & Lau, Y. L. (1993). Disseminated mediastinal carcinoma with chromosomal translocation (15;19). A distinctive clinico-pathologic syndrome. *Cancer, 72,* 2273–2276.

LeRoy, G., Rickards, B., & Flint, S. J. (2008). The double bromodomain proteins Brd2 and Brd3 couple histone acetylation to transcription. *Molecular Cell, 30*, 51–60.

Li, Z., Guo, J., Wu, Y., & Zhou, Q. (2013). The BET bromodomain inhibitor JQ1 activates HIV latency through antagonizing Brd4 inhibition of Tat-transactivation. *Nucleic Acids Research, 41*, 277–287.

Li, G. Q., Guo, W. Z., Zhang, Y., Seng, J. J., Zhang, H. P., Ma, X. X., et al. (2015). Suppression of BRD4 inhibits human hepatocellular carcinoma by repressing MYC and enhancing BIM expression. *Oncotarget, 7*, 2462–2474.

Lockwood, W. W., Zejnullahu, K., Bradner, J. E., & Varmus, H. (2012). Sensitivity of human lung adenocarcinoma cell lines to targeted inhibition of BET epigenetic signaling proteins. *Proceedings of the National Academy of Sciences of the United States of America, 109*, 19408–19413.

Loven, J., Hoke, H. A., Lin, C. Y., Lau, A., Orlando, D. A., Vakoc, C. R., et al. (2013). Selective inhibition of tumor oncogenes by disruption of super-enhancers. *Cell, 153*, 320–334.

Lu, G., Middleton, R. E., Sun, H., Naniong, M., Ott, C. J., Mitsiades, C. S., et al. (2014). The myeloma drug lenalidomide promotes the cereblon-dependent destruction of Ikaros proteins. *Science, 343*, 305–309.

Lupianez, D. G., Kraft, K., Heinrich, V., Krawitz, P., Brancati, F., Klopocki, E., et al. (2015). Disruptions of topological chromatin domains cause pathogenic rewiring of gene-enhancer interactions. *Cell, 161*, 1012–1025.

Maher, O. M., Christensen, A. M., Yedururi, S., Bell, D., & Tarek, N. (2015). Histone deacetylase inhibitor for NUT midline carcinoma. *Pediatric Blood & Cancer, 62*, 715–717.

Mazur, P. K., Herner, A., Mello, S. S., Wirth, M., Hausmann, S., Sanchez-Rivera, F. J., et al. (2015). Combined inhibition of BET family proteins and histone deacetylases as a potential epigenetics-based therapy for pancreatic ductal adenocarcinoma. *Nature Medicine, 21*, 1163–1171.

McCleland, M. L., Mesh, K., Lorenzana, E., Chopra, V. S., Segal, E., Watanabe, C., et al. (2016). CCAT1 is an enhancer-templated RNA that predicts BET sensitivity in colorectal cancer. *The Journal of Clinical Investigation, 126*, 639–652.

Mele, D. A., Salmeron, A., Ghosh, S., Huang, H. R., Bryant, B. M., & Lora, J. M. (2013). BET bromodomain inhibition suppresses TH17-mediated pathology. *The Journal of Experimental Medicine, 210*, 2181–2190.

Mertens, F., Wiebe, T., Adlercreutz, C., Mandahl, N., & French, C. A. (2007). Successful treatment of a child with t(15;19)-positive tumor. *Pediatric Blood & Cancer, 49*, 1015–1017.

Mertz, J. A., Conery, A. R., Bryant, B. M., Sandy, P., Balasubramanian, S., Mele, D. A., et al. (2011). Targeting MYC dependence in cancer by inhibiting BET bromodomains. *Proceedings of the National Academy of Sciences of the United States of America, 108*, 16669–16674.

Muntean, A. G., & Hess, J. L. (2012). The pathogenesis of mixed-lineage leukemia. *Annual Review of Pathology, 7*, 283–301.

Nagoshi, H., Taki, T., Hanamura, I., Nitta, M., Otsuki, T., Nishida, K., et al. (2012). Frequent PVT1 rearrangement and novel chimeric genes PVT1-NBEA and PVT1-WWOX occur in multiple myeloma with 8q24 abnormality. *Cancer Research, 72*, 4954–4962.

Nakamura, Y., Umehara, T., Nakano, K., Jang, M. K., Shirouzu, M., Morita, S., et al. (2007). Crystal structure of the human BRD2 bromodomain: Insights into dimerization and recognition of acetylated histone H4. *The Journal of Biological Chemistry, 282*, 4193–4201.

Nicodeme, E., Jeffrey, K. L., Schaefer, U., Beinke, S., Dewell, S., Chung, C. W., et al. (2010). Suppression of inflammation by a synthetic histone mimic. *Nature, 468*, 1119–1123.

Pivot-Pajot, C., Caron, C., Govin, J., Vion, A., Rousseaux, S., & Khochbin, S. (2003). Acetylation-dependent chromatin reorganization by BRDT, a testis-specific bromodomain-containing protein. *Molecular Cell. Biology, 23*, 5354–5365.

Prinjha, R. K., Witherington, J., & Lee, K. (2012). Place your BETs: The therapeutic potential of bromodomains. *Trends in Pharmacological Sciences, 33*, 146–153.

Puissant, A., Frumm, S. M., Alexe, G., Bassil, C. F., Qi, J., Chanthery, Y. H., et al. (2013). Targeting MYCN in neuroblastoma by BET bromodomain inhibition. *Cancer Discovery, 3*, 308–323.

Qiu, H., Jackson, A. L., Kilgore, J. E., Zhong, Y., Chan, L. L., Gehrig, P. A., et al. (2015). JQ1 suppresses tumor growth through downregulating LDHA in ovarian cancer. *Oncotarget, 6*, 6915–6930.

Rahman, S., Sowa, M. E., Ottinger, M., Smith, J. A., Shi, Y., Harper, J. W., et al. (2011). The Brd4 extraterminal domain confers transcription activation independent of pTEFb by recruiting multiple proteins, including NSD3. *Molecular Cell. Biology, 31*, 2641–2652.

Rathert, P., Roth, M., Neumann, T., Muerdter, F., Roe, J. S., Muhar, M., et al. (2015). Transcriptional plasticity promotes primary and acquired resistance to BET inhibition. *Nature, 525*, 543–547.

Reynoird, N., Schwartz, B. E., Delvecchio, M., Sadoul, K., Meyers, D., Mukherjee, C., et al. (2010). Oncogenesis by sequestration of CBP/p300 in transcriptionally inactive hyperacetylated chromatin domains. *The EMBO Journal, 29*, 2943–2952.

Roe, J. S., Mercan, F., Rivera, K., Pappin, D. J., & Vakoc, C. R. (2015). BET bromodomain inhibition suppresses the function of hematopoietic transcription factors in acute myeloid leukemia. *Molecular Cell, 58*, 1028–1039.

Schroder, S., Cho, S., Zeng, L., Zhang, Q., Kaehlcke, K., Mak, L., et al. (2012). Two-pronged binding with bromodomain-containing protein 4 liberates positive transcription elongation factor b from inactive ribonucleoprotein complexes. *The Journal of Biological Chemistry, 287*, 1090–1099.

Schwartz, B. E., Hofer, M. D., Lemieux, M. E., Bauer, D. E., Cameron, M. J., West, N. H., et al. (2011). Differentiation of NUT midline carcinoma by epigenomic reprogramming. *Cancer Research, 71*, 2686–2696.

Sengupta, S., Biarnes, M. C., Clarke, R., & Jordan, V. C. (2015). Inhibition of BET proteins impairs estrogen-mediated growth and transcription in breast cancers by pausing RNA polymerase advancement. *Breast Cancer Research and Treatment, 150*, 265–278.

Shahbazi, J., Liu, P. Y., Atmadibrata, B., Bradner, J. E., Marshall, G. M., Lock, R. B., et al. (2016). The bromodomain inhibitor JQ1 and the histone deacetylase inhibitor panobinostat synergistically reduce N-Myc expression and induce anticancer effects. *Clinical Cancer Research: An Official Journal of the American Association for Cancer Research.* Epub ahead of print.

Shang, E., Wang, X., Wen, D., Greenberg, D. A., & Wolgemuth, D. J. (2009). Double bromodomain-containing gene Brd2 is essential for embryonic development in mouse. *Developmental Dynamics, 238*, 908–917.

Shehata, B., Steelman, C. K., Abramowsky, C. R., Olson, T., French, C., Saxe, D., et al. (2010). NUT midline carcinoma in a newborn with multiorgan disseminated tumor and a two-year-old with a pancreatic/hepatic primary. *Pediatric and Developmental Pathology, 13*, 481–485.

Shen, C., Ipsaro, J. J., Shi, J., Milazzo, J. P., Wang, E., Roe, J. S., et al. (2015). NSD3-short is an adaptor protein that couples BRD4 to the CHD8 chromatin remodeler. *Molecular Cell, 60*, 847–859.

Shi, J., & Vakoc, C. R. (2014). The mechanisms behind the therapeutic activity of BET bromodomain inhibition. *Molecular Cell, 54*, 728–736.

Shimamura, T., Chen, Z., Soucheray, M., Carretero, J., Kikuchi, E., Tchaicha, J. H., et al. (2013). Efficacy of BET bromodomain inhibition in Kras-mutant non-small cell lung cancer. *Clinical Cancer Research, 19*, 6183–6192.

Shu, S., Lin, C. Y., He, H. H., Witwicki, R. M., Tabassum, D. P., Roberts, J. M., et al. (2016). Response and resistance to BET bromodomain inhibitors in triple-negative breast cancer. *Nature, 529*, 413–417.

Stathis, A., Quesnel, B., Amorim, S., Thieblemont, . C., Zucca, E., Raffoux, E., et al. (2014). 5 LBA: Results of a first-in-man phase I trial assessing OTX015, an orally available BET-bromodomain (BRD) inhibitor, in advanced hematologic malignancies. In *26th EORTC-NCI-AACR symposium on molecular targets and cancer therapeutics: Vol. 50* (pp. 18–21).

Stathis, A., Zucca, E., Bekradda, M., Gomez-Roca, C., Delord, J. P., de La Motte Rouge, T., et al. (2016). Clinical response of carcinomas harboring the BRD4-NUT oncoprotein to the targeted bromodomain inhibitor OTX015/MK-8628. *Cancer Discovery, 6*, 492–500. Epub ahead of print.

Stelow, E. B., Bellizzi, A. M., Taneja, K., Mills, S. E., Legallo, R. D., Kutok, J. L., et al. (2008). NUT rearrangement in undifferentiated carcinomas of the upper aerodigestive tract. *The American Journal of Surgical Pathology, 32*, 828–834.

Stirnweiss, A., McCarthy, K., Oommen, J., Crook, M. L., Hardy, K., Kees, U. R., et al. (2015). A novel BRD4-NUT fusion in an undifferentiated sinonasal tumor highlights alternative splicing as a contributing oncogenic factor in NUT midline carcinoma. *Oncogenesis, 4*, e174.

Stratikopoulos, E. E., Dendy, M., Szabolcs, M., Khaykin, A. J., Lefebvre, C., Zhou, M. M., et al. (2015). Kinase and BET inhibitors together clamp inhibition of pi3k signaling and overcome resistance to therapy. *Cancer Cell, 27*, 837–851.

Stuhlmiller, T. J., Miller, S. M., Zawistowski, J. S., Nakamura, K., Beltran, A. S., Duncan, J. S., et al. (2015). Inhibition of lapatinib-induced kinome reprogramming in ERBB2-positive breast cancer by targeting BET family bromodomains. *Cell Reports, 11*, 390–404.

Suzuki, S., Kurabe, N., Ohnishi, I., Yasuda, K., Aoshima, Y., Naito, M., et al. (2014). NSD3-NUT-expressing midline carcinoma of the lung: First characterization of primary cancer tissue. *Pathology Research and Practice, 211*, 404–408.

Tanaka, M., Kato, K., Gomi, K., Yoshida, M., Niwa, T., Aida, N., et al. (2012). NUT midline carcinoma: Report of 2 cases suggestive of pulmonary origin. *The American Journal of Surgical Pathology, 36*, 381–388.

Thompson-Wicking, K., Francis, R. W., Stirnweiss, A., Ferrari, E., Welch, M. D., Baker, E., et al. (2013). Novel BRD4-NUT fusion isoforms increase the pathogenic complexity in NUT midline carcinoma. *Oncogene, 32*, 4664–4674.

Toretsky, J. A., Jenson, J., Sun, C. C., Eskenazi, A. E., Campbell, A., Hunger, S. P., et al. (2003). Translocation (11;15;19): A highly specific chromosome rearrangement associated with poorly differentiated thymic carcinoma in young patients. *American Journal of Clinical Oncology, 26*, 300–306.

Tseng, Y. Y., Moriarity, B. S., Gong, W., Akiyama, R., Tiwari, A., Kawakami, H., et al. (2014). PVT1 dependence in cancer with MYC copy-number increase. *Nature, 512*, 82–86.

Wang, F., Liu, H., Blanton, W. P., Belkina, A., Lebrasseur, N. K., & Denis, G. V. (2010). Brd2 disruption in mice causes severe obesity without Type 2 diabetes. *The Biochemical Journal, 425*, 71–83.

Winter, G. E., Buckley, D. L., Paulk, J., Roberts, J. M., Souza, A., Dhe-Paganon, S., et al. (2015). DRUG DEVELOPMENT. Phthalimide conjugation as a strategy for in vivo target protein degradation. *Science, 348*, 1376–1381.

Wu, S. Y., Lee, A. Y., Lai, H. T., Zhang, H., & Chiang, C. M. (2013). Phospho switch triggers Brd4 chromatin binding and activator recruitment for gene-specific targeting. *Molecular Cell, 49,* 843–857.

Xiang, J. F., Yin, Q. F., Chen, T., Zhang, Y., Zhang, X. O., Wu, Z., et al. (2014). Human colorectal cancer-specific CCAT1-L lncRNA regulates long-range chromatin interactions at the MYC locus. *Cell Research, 24,* 513–531.

Yan, J., Diaz, J., Jiao, J., Wang, R., & You, J. (2011). Perturbation of BRD4 protein function by BRD4-NUT protein abrogates cellular differentiation in NUT midline carcinoma. *The Journal of Biological Chemistry, 286,* 27663–27675.

Yang, Z., Yik, J. H., Chen, R., He, N., Jang, M. K., Ozato, K., et al. (2005). Recruitment of P-TEFb for stimulation of transcriptional elongation by the bromodomain protein Brd4. *Molecular Cell, 19,* 535–545.

Zhang, W., Prakash, C., Sum, C., Gong, Y., Li, Y., Kwok, J. J., et al. (2012). Bromodomain-containing protein 4 (BRD4) regulates RNA polymerase II serine 2 phosphorylation in human CD4+ T cells. *The Journal of Biological Chemistry, 287,* 43137–43155.

Zhu, J., Gaiha, G. D., John, S. P., Pertel, T., Chin, C. R., Gao, G., et al. (2012). Reactivation of latent HIV-1 by inhibition of BRD4. *Cell Reports, 2,* 807–816.

Zuber, J., Shi, J., Wang, E., Rappaport, A. R., Herrmann, H., Sison, E. A., et al. (2011). RNAi screen identifies Brd4 as a therapeutic target in acute myeloid leukaemia. *Nature, 478,* 524–528.

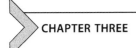
H3K27 Methylation: A Focal Point of Epigenetic Deregulation in Cancer

J.N. Nichol*,1, D. Dupéré-Richer†,1, T. Ezponda‡, J.D. Licht†, W.H. Miller Jr.*,2

*Segal Cancer Centre and Lady Davis Institute, Jewish General Hospital, Division of Experimental Medicine, McGill University, Montreal, QC, Canada
†Division of Hematology Oncology, The University of Florida Health Cancer Center, Gainesville, FL, United States
‡Division of Hematology/Oncology, Centro de Investigacion Medica Aplicada (CIMA), IDISNA, Pamplona, Spain
2Corresponding author: e-mail address: wmiller@ldi.jgh.mcgill.ca

Contents

---

1 These authors contributed equally to this work.

Advances in Cancer Research, Volume 131
ISSN 0065-230X
http://dx.doi.org/10.1016/bs.acr.2016.05.001

Abstract

Epigenetics, the modification of chromatin without changing the DNA sequence itself, determines whether a gene is expressed, and how much of a gene is expressed. Methylation of lysine 27 on histone 3 (H3K27me), a modification usually associated with gene repression, has established roles in regulating the expression of genes involved in lineage commitment and differentiation. Not surprisingly, alterations in the homeostasis of this critical mark have emerged as a recurrent theme in the pathogenesis of many cancers. Perturbations in the distribution or levels of H3K27me occur due to deregulation at all levels of the process, either by mutation in the histone itself, or changes in the activity of the writers, erasers, or readers of this mark. Additionally, as no single histone mark alone determines the overall transcriptional readiness of a chromatin region, deregulation of other chromatin marks can also have dramatic consequences. Finally, the significance of mutations altering H3K27me is highlighted by the poor clinical outcome of patients whose tumors harbor such lesions. Current therapeutic approaches targeting aberrant H3K27 methylation remain to be proven useful in the clinic. Understanding the biological consequences and gene expression pathways affected by aberrant H3K27 methylation may lead to identification of new therapeutic targets and strategies.

1. INTRODUCTION

The transcriptional programs that determine cell fate are stimulus- and cell-type specific. Epigenetic regulation of genes allows different cells to integrate environmental signals with the genetic code to precisely control gene expression and shape cell identity. Epigenetic modifications, namely DNA methylation at CpG sites, and covalent modifications of the N-terminal tails and the core structure of core histones, are critical regulators of chromatin function and help determine accessibility of DNA to the transcription machinery (Kouzarides, 2007). Given the critical role of such modifications in regulating gene expression, it is not surprising that over the past decade, aberrant epigenetic regulation and alteration of histone modifications have emerged as a prominent and recurrent theme in malignancy (Berdasco & Esteller, 2013).

Epigenetic information is deposited by "writer" proteins, such as histone methyl lysine and arginine transferases; removed by "eraser" proteins, such as histone deacetylases and demethylases; and decoded by "reader" proteins adapted to bind to chromatin marks using specific structures, such as the chromo, bromo, and PHD domains (Falkenberg & Johnstone, 2014). The antagonistic activities of two broad classes of protein complexes, trithorax (TrxG) and Polycomb (PcG), are responsible for writing the histone methylation marks that maintain or suppress gene expression. TrxG is associated with activation of gene expression characterized by methylation of lysine 4 of histone H3 (H3K4me), whereas PcG correlated with suppression of gene expression and trimethylation of lysine 27 of histone H3 (H3K27me^3) (Schuettengruber, Martinez, Iovino, & Cavalli, 2011).

In mammals, there are two distinct PcG complexes, PRC1 and PRC2 (Fig. 1). PRC2 is the primary writer of di- and trimethylation of H3K27 which, at certain sites, leads to the recruitment of PRC1. PRC1 ubiqutinates H2A at lysine 119 (H2AK119ub^1), which can then be followed by DNA methyltransferase binding and consequent DNA methylation. Alternatively, H2AK119ub^1 by a variant PRC1 complex can recruit PRC2 de novo, indicating that either PRC1 or PRC2 can initiate a repressive chromatin domain, with recruitment of the other to help maintain or propagate it (Blackledge et al., 2014). PRC2 is composed of four core components, enhancer of zeste homolog 2 (EZH2), suppressor of zeste 12 (SUZ12), and two WD40 domain proteins, EED and RBBP4 (Cao et al., 2002; Muller et al., 2002). The conserved suppressor of variegation,

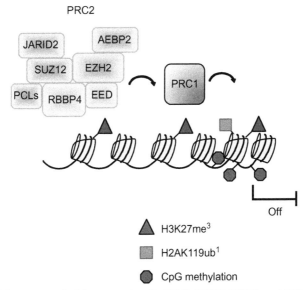

Fig. 1 PRC2 is composed of the core subunits, EZH2, SUZ12, RBBP4, and EED, and is associated with accessory factors, JARID2, AEBP2, and the Polycomb-like proteins (PCLs). PRC2 catalyzes the methylation of histone H3 lysine 27 (H3K27me). PRC1 recognizes, or "reads," the trimethylation of the H3K27 residue (H3K27me^3), a repressive mark, and in turn adds an ubiquitin to histone H2A lysine 119 (H2AK119ub^1). This causes the recruitment of DNA methyltransferases, which will add methyl groups to DNA at CpG islands, and in this way, the repression of chromatin is maintained and propagated. (See the color plate.)

enhancer of zeste, trithorax (SET) domain is the catalytic subunit of EZH2 and has methyltransferase activity not only toward H3K27 but also weakly toward lysine 26 of histone H1 (Kuzmuchev, Nishioka, Erdjument-Bromage, Tempst, & Reinberg, 2002). Early purifications of the PRC2 complex demonstrated that the EZH2 enzyme is active only when associated with EED and SUZ12 and has weak histone methyltransferase activity on its own in vitro (Cao & Zhang, 2004; Czermin et al., 2002; Muller et al., 2002). Thus the noncatalytic subunits have essential roles in regulating the activity and integrity of the complex (Pasini, Bracken, Jensen, Lazzerini Denchi, & Helin, 2004). EZH2 can also interact with histone deacetylases (HDACs) through EED (van der Vlag & Otte, 1999; Zhao et al., 2010) and with noncoding RNA (Jeon & Lee, 2011; van der Vlag & Otte, 1999), thereby providing functional links between the cellular gene repression systems. Other accessory factors including AEBP2 (Cao & Zhang, 2004; Kim, Kang, & Kim, 2009), JARID2 (Li et al., 2010; Peng et al., 2009), and three Polycomb-like proteins (PCLs: PHF1, MTF2, and PHF19) (Boulay, Rosnoblet, Guerardel, Angrand, & Leprince, 2011; Li et al., 2011; Nekrasov et al., 2007; Walker et al., 2010; Zhang, Jones, et al., 2011) have been implicated in the recruitment of PRC2 to its target genes and modulation of its activity. EZH1, a close homolog of EZH2, contains a SET domain, forms an alternative PRC2 complex with SUZ12 and EED, and also catalyzes H3K27 methylation. However, EZH1 and EZH2 exhibit different expression patterns, and the EZH1–PRC2 and EZH2–PRC2 complexes have different methyltransferase and chromatin binding activities (Margueron et al., 2008).

Demethylation of H3K27 is performed by the histone demethylases, UTX/KMD6A and JMJD3/KDM6B, which contain a JmjC (Jumonji) catalytic domain that uses α-ketoglutarate as a cofactor to oxidize and remove the methyl group (Agger et al., 2007; Hong et al., 2007; Lee et al., 2007). UTX interacts with mixed-lineage leukemia (MLL)-containing complexes (Cho et al., 2007; Issaeva et al., 2007; Lee et al., 2007), which are responsible for the activating histone H3 lysine 4 (H3K4) mark, as well as CBP which is a histone acetyl transferase (Tie, Banerjee, Conrad, Scacheri, & Harte, 2012). These results suggest a coordinated mechanism for transcriptional activation, in which repressive H3K27 methyl marks are removed and activating marks are placed.

The amount and distribution of a specific histone modification can be pathologically altered by aberrant expression or function of the writers or erasers, or by mutations of the histone that prevents the residue from being modified. In addition, alterations in the "readers" can mistransduce the signal, thereby altering the functional outcome of the mark. For example, in leukemia, chromosomal translocations involving the plant homeodomain (PHD) fingers of "reader" proteins with the transcriptional activator NUP98, results in inappropriate interpretation of the H3K4 trimethylation mark (H3K4me^3) at genes critical for differentiation (Wang et al., 2009). Finally, histone modifications are intricately coordinated, and alterations of one histone mark can affect the levels and distribution of other modifications. A good example of this *trans*-regulation is the stimulation of SET1-dependent H3K4me$^{2/3}$ by histone H2B (H2B) ubiquitination (Kim, Bird, et al., 2013).

Given the wealth of evidence of the importance of H3K27me in the pathogenesis of cancer, in this review we will focus on mechanisms that affect the levels and distribution of this mark in human malignancies.

2. HISTONE H3 MUTATIONS

The human histone H3 family of proteins consists of seven members, the two "canonical" H3, H3.1 and H3.2, and five variants, H3.3, CENP-A, H3t (Witt, Albig, & Doenecke, 1996), H3.X, and H3.Y (Wiedemann et al., 2010). Histone proteins are decorated by a variety of protein posttranslational modifications (PTMs), which are critical to dynamic modulation of chromatin structure and function and contribute to the cellular gene expression program. As with canonical H3, histone tails of the variants are still subject to PTMs.

Recurrent, cancer-driving mutations are found in the genes encoding histones. Specifically, sequencing studies in pediatric and young adult high-grade gliomas have identified somatic missense mutations of histone H3 that results in a lysine 27 to methionine change (H3K27M) (Schwartzentruber et al., 2012; Sturm et al., 2012; Wu, Broniscer, et al., 2012). The majority of K27M mutations have been found in the gene encoding H3.3, *H3F3A*, with a few occurrences in genes that encode canonical H3, *HIST1H3B* and *HIST1H3C* (Buczkowicz et al., 2014; Fontebasso et al., 2014; Khuong-Quang et al., 2012; Schwartzentruber et al., 2012; Sturm et al., 2012; Wu, Broniscer, et al., 2012). The K27M mutations in H3 are predictors of poor survival (Khuong-Quang et al., 2012; Sturm et al., 2012).

Histone H3.3 deposition is the result of the replacement of histone H3 (normally incorporated into chromatin during S phase) with the variant, which is incorporated outside S phase at particular loci (Ahmad &

Henikoff, 2002). H3.3 is enriched at pericentromeric and telomeric regions (Szenker, Ray-Gallet, & Almouzni, 2011), and importantly, at transcriptionally "active" or "poised" regions of the genome (Goldberg et al., 2010). H3.3's pronounced patterns of genomic enrichment are mediated by at least two independent histone chaperones, with HIRA mainly facilitating deposition at gene loci (Ray-Gallet et al., 2002) and ATRX/DAXX responsible for repeat regions (Lewis, Elsaesser, Noh, Stadler, & Allis, 2010). The poised regions into which histone H3.3 is placed are enriched for lysine 4 trimethylation of H3 (H3K4me^3), or for both lysine 27 trimethylation (H3K27me^3) and H3K4me^3 (Delbarre et al., 2010). Thus the deposition of mutant histones could perturb the delicate balance of histone modifications in these crucial regions.

In vitro evidence suggests that the mutations act in a dominant negative manner by directly inhibiting PRC2 methyltransferase activity (Bender et al., 2013; Lewis et al., 2013) and "trap" or "poison" the PRC2 complex. In doing so, the mutant histones prevent the deposition of methyl marks on other PRC2 target regions, and thus can affect the entirety of the cellular transcriptional program. In support of this, chromatin immunoprecipitation sequencing (ChIP-Seq) analysis of cultured glioma cells with the H3.3K27M mutation measured fewer H3K27me^3 peaks compared to controls (Bender et al., 2013; Chan et al., 2013), but interestingly, the lower abundance was not uniform over the genome. Instead, there was a genomic redistribution of H3K27me^3 marks, with increases and decreases in gene expression corresponding to decreases and increases in local H3K27me^3 levels, respectively. An innovative model of diffuse intrinsic pontine glioma (DIPG) was created by differentiating human embryonic stem (ES) cells into neural progenitor cells and then transducing them with a viral vector to force expression of H3.3K27M (Funato, Major, Lewis, Allis, & Tabar, 2014). This study by Funato and colleagues demonstrated that expression of H3.3K27M alone is insufficient to confer features of neoplastic cells, but it does synergize with other common DIPG gene alterations, in this case p53 loss and PDGFRA activation, to cause oncogenic transformation (Funato et al., 2014). The same study showed that H3.3K27M-induced mitogenic stimulation was restricted to neural progenitors, with no effect seen in undifferentiated ES cells or astrocytes, suggesting that the histone mutation is oncogenic only within the appropriate developmental window. An overlapping analysis of gene expression patterns and chromatin modifications showed that H3.3K27M expression promoted dedifferentiation to a more primitive, stem-like state (Funato et al., 2014). Additionally, studies have demonstrated codependency between DNA methylation and histone H3K27me^3 patterns (Brinkman et al., 2012; Statham et al., 2012), and the overall reductions in DNA methylation seen in patient samples with H3.3K27M (Bender et al., 2013; Sturm et al., 2012) may work in concert with the mutated histone to help stabilize the tumor phenotype.

Mutations of other histone residues may also indirectly affect H3K27me^3. A significant proportion of chondroblastoma and giant cell bone tumors have a mutation of lysine 36 of histone H3 to a methionine (K36M) (Behjati et al., 2013). Similar to the K27M mutants, K36M mutants display global reductions in H3K36 methylation. H3K36me$^{2/3}$ and H3K27me$^{2/3}$ marks are mutually exclusive (Yuan et al., 2011; Zheng et al., 2012), and thus, the reduction of H3K36me levels observed with K36M mutants may remove a damper on PRC2 activity, resulting in expansion of the H3K27me^3 mark and aberrant repression of many loci. However, further research is needed to determine the nature of genes deregulated in such tumors.

Finally, altering the epigenetic landscape may not be the only mechanism by which histone H3 mutants affect gene expression programs. Mutation of the N-terminal tail could alter recognition of H3.3 by chromatin-remodeling enzymes or chaperones, such as DAXX (Lewis et al., 2010), that may disrupt normal incorporation of H3.3 in pericentromeric regions. This in turn could affect chromosomal segregation, as was observed when H3.3 levels were knocked-down (Bush et al., 2013; Lin, Conti, & Ramalho-Santos, 2013). Additionally, these mutations could affect H3.3 turnover kinetics or induce conformational changes that disrupt normal chromatin architecture. Thus, histone H3 mutants might disrupt the cytogenetic integrity of a cell, changes which might facilitate carcinogenesis.

3. ALTERATIONS IN H3K27me "WRITERS"

3.1 EZH2 Overexpression

Accumulating evidence suggests that *EZH2* acts as an oncogene and its aberrant overexpression has been documented in both solid tumors and hematological malignancies. Amplification of EZH2 (Bracken et al., 2003; Saramaki, Tammela, Martikainen, Vessella, & Visakorpi, 2006) and alterations in microRNA levels have been proposed as the cause of EZH2 deregulation (Friedman et al., 2009; Kong et al., 2012; Varambally et al., 2008).

Overexpression of EZH2 in chronic lymphocytic leukemia patients correlates with important indicators of poor prognosis, including high white blood cell counts, ZAP-70 expression, and chromosomal abnormalities (Rabello Ddo et al., 2015). Overexpression was also reported in patients with high-risk myelodysplastic syndrome (MDS), MDS-derived acute myeloid leukemia (AML), and AML, particularly in patients with complex karyotypes and correlates with levels of DNA methylation and poor prognostic scoring (Grubach et al., 2008; Xu et al., 2011). Overexpression of EZH2 itself is insufficient to cause leukemia, but does prevent hematopoietic stem cell (HSC) exhaustion (Kamminga et al., 2006). When EZH2 was knocked out in the MLL-AF9 mouse model of AML, growth of leukemic cells was compromised in vitro and leukemia progression slowed in vivo (Tanaka et al., 2012). In this model, EZH2 represses genes relevant to differentiation, apoptosis, and stem cell function, such as EGR1, and reduces leukemia-initiating cell frequency. However, the results of this model, where the leukemia induced is produced via perturbation of another histone methyltransferase, MLL1, complicates interpretation of the results and makes it difficult to delineate a role for EZH2 alone.

EZH2 is aberrantly overexpressed in a majority of natural killer/T-cell lymphoma (NKTL), as gene expression profiling (GEP) of formalin-fixed, paraffin-embedded tissues showed overexpression of EZH2 compared to normal NK cells (Ng et al., 2011). The overexpression is due to MYC suppression of microRNAs that normally target and inhibit EZH2 expression.

In solid tumors, high levels of EZH2 are clinically associated with aggressive biology, metastasis, and poor clinical outcome (Bachmann et al., 2006; Kleer et al., 2003; Sasaki, Yamaguchi, Itatsu, Ikeda, & Nakanuma, 2008; Varambally et al., 2002). Similarly, in model cell lines, overexpression of EZH2 promotes anchorage-independent growth and cell invasion, and correlates with cancer progression (Kleer et al., 2003; Xu et al., 2012).

Traditional thinking dictates that overexpressed EZH2 exerts its oncogenic activity via its SET domain, and presumably, its ability to mark histones for gene repression. Indeed, EZH2 overexpression has been linked to increased H3K27me^3 levels and repression of tumor suppressor genes (Kim & Yu, 2012; Wang et al., 2012). In line with these findings, GEP of human melanoma patients identified a new set of EZH2 target genes that when expressed at low levels, correlated poorly with survival. Importantly, these target genes displayed tumor-suppressive functions affecting either melanoma growth or metastatic spread (Zingg et al., 2015).

However, evidence suggests that EZH2 has potential functions other than that of a transcriptional repressor, although potential mechanisms remain incompletely characterized. In NKTL, EZH2 behaves unconventionally in

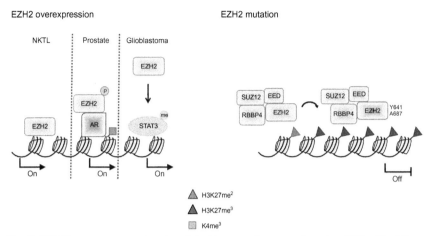

Fig. 2 EZH2 is overexpressed and mutated in several cancers. In natural killer/T-cell lymphoma (NKTL), prostate cancer and glioblastoma, overexpression of EZH2 causes it to have activities beyond H3K27 methylation (*left panel*). In diffuse large B-cell lymphoma (DLBCL), common mutations in EZH2 increases the enzyme's efficiency, resulting in an increase in H3K27me^3 levels. These mutations are heterozygous and work with the wild-type EZH2 (*right panel*). (See the color plate.)

that its promotion of growth is independent of its SET domain (ie, methyltransferase activity), and it serves as a transcriptional activator, by binding to and positively regulating the *CCND1* promoter (Yan et al., 2013). In prostate cancer cell lines (Xu et al., 2012), phosphorylated EZH2 did not associate with the PRC2 complex, but bound the androgen receptor, and was present at actively transcribed genes. This activity did require the SET domain of EZH2, suggesting that methylation of nonhistone targets may also be relevant for the oncogenic action of EZH2. In support of the idea that nonhistone targets are important mediators of EZH2 action, in glioblastoma, phosphorylated EZH2 methylates STAT3, increasing the activation of this oncogenic transcription factor (Kim, Kim, et al., 2013) (Fig. 2).

3.2 EZH2 Mutations

Just as overexpression of EZH2 has pathological consequences, mutations in EZH2, both activating and inactivating, are found in a variety of tumors.

Non-Hodgkin's lymphoma is a heterogeneous disease with frequent mutations in histone-modifying enzymes. In 2010, next-generation sequencing identified heterozygous somatic missense mutations in 7% of follicular lymphoma (FL) and in up to 22% of diffuse large B-cell lymphoma

(DLBCL) cases (Morin et al., 2010). Notably, the DLBCL patients that were positive for *EZH2* mutations, were of the germinal center B-cell like (GCB), and not the activated B-cell-like molecular subtype. The mutations are found within the SET domain of EZH2 at tyrosine 641 (Y64N, F, S, or H) (Morin et al., 2010), alanine 677 (A677G) (McCabe et al., 2012), and alanine 687 (A687V) (Majer et al., 2012).

The Y641 mutant can be incorporated into the PRC2 complex, and it was initially reported to be a loss-of-function (LOF) mutation (Morin et al., 2010). Subsequent work however demonstrated a gain-of-function (GOF) for the mutant, whereby the mutant EZH2 has minimal activity for $H3K27me^0$ and $H3K27me^1$, but has enhanced catalytic efficiency for the $H3K27me^2$ to $H3K27me^3$ conversion. The fact that all the Y641 mutations are heterozygous implies that the malignant phenotype of disease requires the coordinated activities of the wild-type (WT) EZH2, to monomethylate H3K27, and the mutant EZH2, for increased conversion of H3K27 to the trimethylated form (Sneeringer et al., 2010; Yap et al., 2011). EZH2 A687V works similarly to the Y641 mutations (Majer et al., 2012). In contrast, EZH2 A677G has equal affinity for all three methylation substrates ($H3K27me^0$, $H3K27me^1$, and $H3K27me^2$) (Majer et al., 2012; McCabe et al., 2012; Wu, Northcott, et al., 2012).

In lymphoma, the end result of all documented mutations is elevated global H3K27 trimethylation, constitutive repression of genes required for B-cell differentiation, and an expansion of B-cells at the germinal center stage that can ultimately lead to malignancy (Beguelin et al., 2013) (Fig. 2). The recurrent mutations in EZH2 make it an attractive therapeutic target in B-cell malignancies. Indeed, small-molecule inhibitors of EZH2 function (EZH2i) have been developed that show potent inhibition of DLBCL-cell line proliferation in vitro. The clinical targeting of EZH2 in DLBCL and other malignancies is discussed in more detail in Section 7.

Paradoxically, evidence in leukemia suggests that it is the loss of EZH2 that contributes to tumor development. In T-cell acute lymphoblastic leukemia (T-ALL), myeloproliferative disorders and myeloid malignancies, a range of missense, nonsense, and frameshift mutations of *EZH2* occur (Ernst et al., 2010; Nikoloski et al., 2010; Ntziachristos et al., 2012). These lesions can be heterozygous or homozygous, are found throughout the gene body, and generally are predicted to ablate HMT activity via truncation of the SET domain. Loss of EZH2 potentiates oncogenic NOTCH1 and RUNX1 signaling in T-ALL and MDS, respectively (Ntziachristos et al., 2012; Sashida et al., 2014). Loss of EZH2 is an indicator of poor prognosis in MDS (Ernst et al., 2010; Nikoloski et al., 2010), but the same association with de novo AML cannot be drawn, as EZH2 mutations remain comparatively rare in this setting (Wang et al., 2013). While MDS may often convert to AML, this does not to be the case for MDS associated with EZH2 loss, suggesting that such patients succumb to progressive pancytopenia rather than leukemic progression.

In contrast to the wealth of data describing EZH2 mutations in a hematopoietic setting, the role of EZH2 mutations in solid malignancies remains relatively uncharacterized. EZH2 Y641 mutations have recently been identified in roughly 2% of human melanomas (Hodis et al., 2012). Ectopic expression of EZH2 GOF mutations in a melanoma cell line resulted in increased H3K27me^3 and dramatic changes in 3D culture morphology in vitro and larger tumor size in vivo (Barsotti et al., 2015). Sequencing of head and neck squamous cell carcinoma patient's tumors revealed the presence inactivating mutations in EZH2 (Stransky et al., 2011), although many other studies suggest that EZH2 acts as an oncogene in HNSCC cell lines (Gannon, Merida de Long, Endo-Munoz, Hazar-Rethinam, & Saunders, 2013).

The fact that LOF and GOF EZH2 mutations occur in cancer implies binary, tissue-specific roles for the protein as both oncogene and tumor suppressor and highlights the importance of the balance of this histone mark for cell homeostasis.

3.3 Mutations in Polycomb Group-Associated Proteins

Efficient H3K27 methylation requires the cooperation of several PRC2 core components in addition to EZH2, specifically SUZ12 and EED. Knockout of either of these genes in ES cells results in severe global reduction of H3K27me^3 (Pasini, Bracken, Hansen, Capillo, & Helin, 2007). SUZ12 and EED are found mutated in several cancers, like nerve sheath tumors (Lee et al., 2014), myeloproliferative neoplasms (MPN) (Brecqueville et al., 2011), and early T-cell T-ALL (Zhang et al., 2012). In some of them decreased in H3K27me^3 was observed. The PRC2 complex recognizes the product of its own catalysis, H3K27me$^{2/3}$, through its EED subunit, leading to a stimulation of its methyltransferase activity (Xu et al., 2010). Therefore, as EED serves as a reader for H3K27me$^{2/3}$, we consider it in the following Section 4.

JARID2, a more recently identified PRC2-associated protein, is important for recruiting both PRC1 and PRC2 to promoters (Pasini, Cloos, et al.,

2010). However, its role in directly regulating H3K27 methylation remains uncertain. JARID2 is not required for maintaining global H3K27 methylation, although it does participate in maintaining this mark at selected promoters. In T–ALL and MDS, rare missense mutations in JARID2 were found (Score et al., 2012; Simon et al., 2012), but were not predicted to be inactivating, and therefore the relevance of these mutations in H3K27me^3 patterning is unclear.

Mimicking the loss of EZH2 in MDS, MPN, and myeloid malignancies, recurrent somatic mutations and deletions of *ASXL1*, which encodes another PRC2-associated factor (Abdel-Wahab et al., 2012), result in loss of PRC2-mediated H3K27me^3. As a result, many genes are aberrantly activated, including the *HOXA* cluster, contributing to myeloid transformation and inducement of an MDS-like disease in mice (Abdel-Wahab et al., 2012; Inoue et al., 2013).

4. ALTERATIONS IN H3K27me "READERS"

The chromodomain of "reader" proteins recognizes methylation marks on histones. With the help of WD40 domains that recruit effector molecules, chromodomains determine the propagation and maintenance of a silent chromatin conformation. Aberrations in chromodomain proteins are commonly found in cancer and lead to misinterpretation of the chromatin state (Fig. 3).

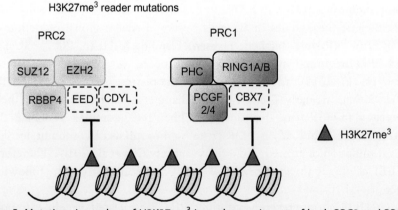

Fig. 3 Mutations in readers of H3K27me^3 impede recruitment of both PRC2 and PRC1 complexes, which prevents the maintenance and/or propagation of a silent chromatin state. (See the color plate.)

The chromodomain protein CDYL binds H3K27me^3 and recruits EZH2, bridging the PRC2 complex to chromatin. CDYL's interaction with H3K27me^3 enhances PRC2 methyltransferase activity and thus, creates a positive feedback loop that helps to maintain chromatin in a silent state (Zhang, Yang, et al., 2011). CDYL loss of heterozygosity is found in cervical cancer and is associated with poor prognosis. The decreased expression in CDYL was shown to derepress the proto-oncogene *NTRK3* and to lead to oncogenic transformation in vitro (Mulligan et al., 2008). Likewise, the chromodomain of CDYL, and its homolog CDYL2, exhibit missense and nonsense mutations that could impact their ability to recognize methylation marks on chromatin (Cerami et al., 2012; Gao et al., 2013).

CBX (Chromobox Homolog) proteins are responsible for the recruitment of the PRC1 complex at specific loci by recognizing H3K27me marks. PRC1 will further create a silent chromatin conformation by methylating H3K9. In many cancer types, loss of CBX7 expression is associated with invasiveness and epithelial-to-mesenchymal transition (EMT) (Federico et al., 2009; Forzati et al., 2012; Karamitopoulou et al., 2010; Pallante et al., 2014). However, CBX7 was also shown to act as an oncogene. Overexpression of CBX7 in hematopoietic stem progenitor cells enhances self-renewal and induces leukemia, an effect that requires a functional chromodomain (Klauke et al., 2013).

Although EED does not possess a chromodomain, some residues in its WD40 domain form a pocket interacting with H3K27me (Margueron et al., 2009). One rare mutation in the WD40 motif was shown to inhibit its interaction with H3K27me^3, and global H3K27me^3 is severely impaired in the cells overexpressing this mutant (Ueda et al., 2012). The most frequent mutations in EED seem to disrupt the formation of PRC2 and abrogate the H3K27 methyltransferase activity of PRC2 (Denisenko, Shnyreva, Suzuki, & Bomsztyk, 1998; Khan et al., 2013; Score et al., 2012).

Methylation of H3K27 can also inhibit binding of effector molecules. AF10 and AF17 recognize unmodified H3K27 through a PHD finger–Zn knuckle–PHD finger (PZP) module and this is required for DOT1L-mediated H3K79 methylation and gene expression (Chen et al., 2015). Of note, *AF10* and *AF17* are involved in recurrent chromosomal translocations with MLL in leukemia, making these tumors addicted to DOT1L (Chen et al., 2015; Deshpande et al., 2014). PZP-mediated interaction between AF10 and H3K27 plays a critical role in regulating both the expression of DOT1L-target genes and the proliferation of DOT1L-addicted leukemic cells. However, the binding to H3K27 by AF10-containing oncofusions has not been investigated.

Aberrations in readers of H3K27me^3 can therefore contribute to outcomes as dramatic as the ones caused by deregulation of chromatin writers and erasers. However, more work is needed to better characterize the mechanisms of action of these mutations.

5. ALTERATIONS IN H3K27 "ERASERS"

The H3K27 methylation mark may be removed by the UTX (KDM6A) and JMJD3 (KMD6B) proteins, both containing the jumonji domains and using an oxidation-based mechanism of removing the methyl residues. In both hematological malignancies and solid tumors, disruption of H3K27 demethylase activity via mutation of *UTX* is far more common in cancer patients than disruption due to *JMJD3* mutations (Gui et al., 2011; Statham et al., 2012; Van der Meulen et al., 2015; van Haaften et al., 2009). However, a subset of glioblastoma multiforme patients does have somatic mutations of *JMJD3*, or downregulation of its mRNA expression secondary to DNA hypermethylation (Ene et al., 2012; Monti et al., 2012). Furthermore, cases of FL that have transformed to large cell lymphoma may suffer from inactivating mutations of JMJD3, which are mutually exclusive from KMT2D/MLL2 mutations (Carlotti et al., 2015).

Several recent whole-genome sequencing studies of bladder cancer patients revealed that *UTX* was inactivated in about 25% cases (Guo et al., 2013; Nickerson et al., 2014; Waddell et al., 2015). Exome sequencing also revealed a significant frequency of *UTX* mutations in pancreatic tumors and GEP revealed that the mutations were enriched in a subtype in which p53 mutations were also enriched, and that subtype had a poorer prognosis (Bailey et al., 2016). *UTX* is located on the X-chromosome and the mutations are homozygous in females and hemizygous in males (van Haaften et al., 2009). However, in males, loss of UTX was accompanied by loss of UTX's paralog located on the Y chromosome, *UTY* (van Haaften et al., 2009).

As with EZH2, UTX behaves paradoxically, and both tumor suppressor and oncogenic effects are seen with alterations in UTX. In some models, loss of UTX enhances the proliferation of cancer cells (Ho et al., 2013; Van der Meulen et al., 2015; van Haaften et al., 2009) and in others, UTX overexpression promotes proliferation (Kim et al., 2014). The effect is not tissue specific, as in breast cancer UTX expression is associated with invasion and clinically, high levels of UTX are associated with poor prognosis in patients (Kim et al., 2014). However, UTX expression also plays an important role in breast tumor suppression by silencing transcription factors important in the EMT (Choi et al., 2015). In these cases, the confusion concerning UTX's role may be attributed to its partner at the time (KMT2D vs LSD1/HDAC1) or whether the activity is H3K27me-demethylase dependent or independent.

Finally, the mutual exclusivity of *UTX* mutations with other genes might provide clues as to UTX's place in essential biological pathways in different tissues. For example, inactivating mutations of UTX and the H3K4 methyltransferase, KMT2D (Nickerson et al., 2014) in bladder cancer are mutually exclusive. Expression of some UTX-modulated genes is also regulated by the H3K4 methyltransferase KMT2D, whose C-terminal region interacts with UTX (Kim et al., 2014). The mutual exclusivity seen with these two proteins suggests a functional redundancy and that they cooperatively regulate gene expression programs. In multiple myeloma (MM), UTX null samples are all negative for the MMSET-activating t(4;14) translocation (van Haaften et al., 2009). Together, these findings indicate that balances in H3K27/H3K4 and H3K27/H3K36 methylation are critical for cell homeostasis.

6. CROSS TALK WITH OTHER CHROMATIN REGULATORS

The discovery that chromatin modifiers were heavily mutated in all cancers paved the way for studies attempting to understand the interplay between the epigenetic modifiers and histone modifications affected by these mutations. Many histone-modifying enzymes involved in the pathogenesis of cancer indirectly impact on H3K27me level genome wide and at specific locus.

6.1 MMSET Overexpression

In MM harboring the t(4;14) translocation, the H3K36-specific HMT, MMSET/NSD2 is fused to the immunoglobulin heavy-chain locus, leading to MMSET overexpression (Keats et al., 2005). This genetic aberration is associated with poor prognosis (Keats et al., 2003), and the increase in MMSET expression was shown to drive cell proliferation, clonogenecity, and invasion of MM cells (Brito et al., 2009; Ezponda et al., 2013; Kuo et al., 2011; Lauring et al., 2008; Martinez-Garcia et al., 2011). Overexpression of MMSET causes a genome wide increase in H3K36me^2, concomitant with a global reduction in H3K27me^3 (Fig. 4A) (Ezponda et al., 2013). However, some specific loci were shielded from the effects of the

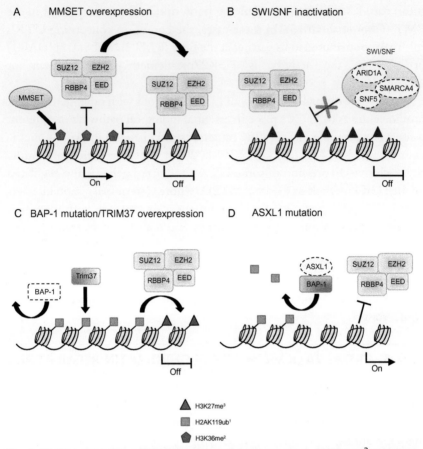

Fig. 4 (A) Overexpression of MMSET induces global increases in H3K36me^2, which prevents its recognition by PRC2. Therefore, PRC2 accumulates at specific loci, where it binds chromatin and represses transcription. (B) Through modulation of nucleosome density, the chromatin remodeling complex SWI/SNF prevents methylation of H3K27 by PRC2. The many mutations in SWI/SNF subunits inactivate its activity and lead to increased levels of H3K27me^3. (C) H2A ubiquitination increases PRC2 affinity for nucleosomes, which leads to increased H3K27me^3. The inactivation of the DUB enzyme, BAP-1, and overexpression of the ubiquitinase TRIM37 favors global increases in H3K27me^3 and silencing of chromatin. (D) On the other hand, mutated ASXL1 enhances the DUB activity of BAP-1, leading to decreased levels of H3K27me^3 with gene activation. (See the color plate.)

overexpressed MMSET and exhibited high H3K27me^3 levels with increased EZH2 binding, leading to repression of transcription of such loci (Popovic et al., 2012). Thus, MMSET overexpression simultaneously leads to global decreases, but local increases in H3K27me^3, suggesting that a few genes are mediating the oncogenic effect. Consistent with this hypothesis, cells expressing high levels of MMSET are more sensitive to molecules inhibiting EZH2 (Popovic et al., 2012), and this correlates with activation of the specific loci-repressed genes. Therefore, H3K27me^3-mediated repression of some genes is relevant to the molecular pathogenesis of this form of malignancy.

A similar interplay between H3K36me and H3K27me was observed in other malignancies. In pediatric B-cell ALL (B-ALL) and mantle cell lymphoma, a recurrent mutation within the catalytic SET domain of MMSET mimics the effects of MMSET overexpression on cell growth and was similarly able to induce a global increase in H3K36me^2 concomitantly with a genome-wide decrease in H3K27me^3 (Bea et al., 2013; Jaffe et al., 2013; Oyer et al., 2014). Furthermore, the t(5;11) translocation found in AML, leading to fusion of the MMSET homolog *NSD1*, and *NUP98* was shown to cause local increases in H3K36me^2 simultaneously with loss of EZH2 and H3K27me^3 at the *HOXA* locus. This effect was associated with the transforming properties of NUP98-NSD1 and required NSD1 HMT activity (Wang, Cai, Pasillas, & Kamps, 2007).

EZH2 and MMSET expression are tightly correlated in cancers, and EZH2 function was suggested to be required for MMSET activity. In fact, EZH2 regulates MMSET expression by attenuating the expression micro-RNAs, such as miR-203, miR-26a, and miR-31, and indirectly cause increase H3K36me^2. Furthermore, EZH2 neoplastic properties were shown to require MMSET expression (Asangani et al., 2013; Ezponda et al., 2013).

6.2 SWI/SNF Chromatin-Remodeling Complex Inactivation

The SWI/SNF chromatin-remodeling complex antagonizes the PRC2 complex activity at its target genes (Kia, Gorski, Giannakopoulos, & Verrijzer, 2008). SWI/SNF is frequently inactivated in cancer, most notably in rhabdoid tumors, where almost all cases present with a mutation in one of the SWI/SNF complex subunits. It was hypothesized that nucleosome density, which is regulated by SWI/SNF, affects PRC2 activity and deposition of methylation on H3K27 (Yuan et al., 2012). For instance, loss of SNF5, also found in T-cell lymphoma, decreases polycomb protein displacement at specific loci leading to an increase in EZH2 and H3K27me^3 (Fig. 4B) (Wilson et al., 2010). This causes the repression of genes critical for differentiation and tumor suppression such as *HOXB1* (Wilson et al., 2010) and *CDKN2A* (Kia et al., 2008). *ARID1A* encodes a component of the SWI/SNF chromatin-remodeling complex that is also frequently mutated in many tumors (Lawrence et al., 2014), including ovarian clear cell carcinoma (OCCC). Inhibition of EZH2 reduced overall H3K27me^3 levels in both wild-type and *ARID1A*-mutated OCCC cells, while selectively suppressing proliferation of *ARID1A*-mutated cell lines, suggesting that H3K27me^3 at specific loci drives tumorigenesis. Indeed, EZH2 inhibitor (EZH2i) selectivity toward ARID1A-mutated tumors was associated with increased PIK3IP1 expression and decreased AKT activation (Bitler et al., 2015). Overall, these studies suggest that SWI/SNF-inactivated tumors depend on PRC2-mediated H3K27me^3 at specific genes. However, non-SET activity may be also important, as one study demonstrated that SWI/SNF-mutated cancer cells were dependent on both catalytic and non-catalytic activity of EZH2 and this was abolished by the presence of mutations in RAS pathway (Kim et al., 2015).

6.3 Histone Acetylation

Lysine K27 on H3 can also be targeted by acetylation, and this modification is mutually exclusive with methylation (Tie et al., 2009; Pasini, Malatesta, et al., 2010). The acetyltransferases CBP/p300 catalyze this reaction and consequently, antagonize the methylation and repression of transcription by PRC2 (Pasini, Malatesta, et al., 2010). HDACs catalyze the reverse reaction. HDAC1 and HDAC3 interact with PRC2 complex (van der Vlag & Otte, 1999) and promote H3K27me by removing acetylation on H3K27, thus making lysine 27 on H3 free for subsequent methylation by EZH2. Indeed, ablation or inhibition of PRC2 promotes H3K27ac genome wide and also at specific loci such as proximal promoter and enhancers (Pasini, Malatesta, et al., 2010; Xu et al., 2015).

CBP/p300 is inactivated in about 30% cases of DLBCL (Pasqualucci et al., 2011) and in 18% of cases of ALL, raising the possibility that PRC2-regulated genes are maintained in a repressed state in these cancers. However, no studies have examined the effect of histone acetyltransferase (HAT) inactivation on the regulation of PRC2 target genes. HDAC expression is increased in various cancers (Adams, Fritzsche, Dirnhofer, Kristiansen, & Tzankov, 2010; Choi et al., 2001; Marquard et al., 2008; Wada et al., 2009; Zhang et al., 2005), and inhibitors of HDAC activity have been shown to decrease global H3K27me3 (Fiskus et al., 2006). HDAC inhibitors also markedly attenuated EZH2-mediated invasion of cancer cell lines (Cao et al., 2008). Moreover, a correlation was established between HDAC1 and H3K27me^3 occupancy genome wide and the correlation was more significant at promoter regions (Song et al., 2015). Overall, these data show that HDAC/HAT activity is determinant in establishing H3K27me^3 marks throughout the genome.

6.4 Wilms' Tumor 1 Mutations

Wilms' tumor 1 (WT1) is a transcription factor harboring inactivating mutations within its DNA-binding zinc finger domain in about 10% of AML cases. WT1 interacts with the enzyme-mediating DNA demethylation, TET2, to regulate its target genes (Wang et al., 2015). Consequently, the loss of *WT1* was associated with global increase in DNA methylation (Rampal et al., 2014), and hypermethylated genes were shown to strongly overlap with genes targeted by PRC2/H3K27me, leading to aberrant repression of H3K27me-marked gene in WT1 mutant tumors (Sinha et al., 2015). Moreover, inhibition of EZH2 is able to induce a better myeloid differentiation response in WT1 mutant than in WT1 wild-type primary acute promyelocytic leukemia.

6.5 MLL Oncofusions

The H3K4-specific HMT, MLL (MLL1/KMT2A), is frequently rearranged with a large number of varied genes in AML and this is associated with poor prognosis (Behm et al., 1996). All fusion oncoproteins involving MLL have lost HMT activity, but still recruit coactivators of transcription, epigenetic modifiers, including DOT1L, and together aberrantly induce transcription of oncogenes like *MYC*, *MEIS1*, and *HOX*, and also *EZH2*. Even though the genome-wide pattern of H3K27me in MLL-rearranged leukemias has not yet been investigated, these tumors have been shown to depend on PRC2 activity to promote growth and self-renewal of leukemia (Neff et al., 2012; Shi et al., 2013). Furthermore, they exhibit sensitivity toward inhibition of both EZH1 and EZH2 enzymes, and this is associated with decreased H3K27me^3 at enhancers and promoters of specific genes related to development and differentiation (Xu et al., 2015). Inhibition of PRC2 only minimally affects the expression of well-established direct target genes of MLL-AF9, which also harbor minimal levels of H3K27 methylation at their promoters (Shi et al., 2013). This is consistent with the fact that methylation of H3K27 inhibits recruitment of the MLL-fusion interacting partner, AF10 (Chen et al., 2015). Together these results suggest that MLL-fusions and PRC2 target distinct site in the genome and act complementary in promoting tumorigenesis.

6.6 H2A Monoubiquitination

H3K27me^3 can direct the recruitment of the PRC1 complex to chromatin. PRC1 possesses E3 ubiquitin ligase activity toward H2AK119. Monoubiquitinated H2AK119 (H2AK119ub^1) can in turn recruit PRC2 complex to maintain chromatin in a repressed conformation. H2AK119ub[1] increases the affinity of the PRC2 complex to nucleosomes and is sufficient to drive H3K27me[3] deposition, although the mechanism by which this occurs is still undefined (Blackledge et al., 2014; Kalb et al., 2014). Inversely, UTX-mediated demethylation of H3K27 reduces the recruitment of the canonical PRC1 complex and consequently, will decrease H2A mono-ubiquitination (Lee et al., 2007).

In cancer, perturbations in this relationship can favor the increases in H3K27me[3] (Fig. 4C). The ubiquitin ligase TRIM37 catalyzes H2AK119ub[1]. This gene is amplified in about 40% of breast cancers and this is associated with decreased survival of estrogen-receptor positive patients. TRIM37-targeted gene promoters were shown to recruit PRC2 and exhibited high levels of H3K27me[3] and transcriptional silencing. Furthermore, knockdown of *TRIM37* reversed these events (Bhatnagar et al., 2014). The deubiquitinating (DUB) enzyme targeting H2AK119ub[1], BRCA1-associated protein-1 (BAP-1), is a tumor suppressor inactivated in a variety of malignancies (Dey et al., 2012; Harbour et al., 2010; Pena-Llopis et al., 2012; Testa et al., 2011). BAP-1 loss was shown to transform cells in an EZH2-dependent manner, leading to a global increase in H3K27me[3] (LaFave et al., 2015). Interestingly, BAP-1 mutations cooccur with UTX mutations in bladder cancer, which suggest that these factors may have complementary functions in driving tumorigenesis (Nickerson et al., 2014). These data suggest that deregulation of enzymes meditating H2AK119ub[1] in cancer may lead to outcomes similar to EZH2 overexpression.

Conversely, the deregulation of enzymes regulating H2AK119ub[1] levels can tip the scale against H3K27 methylation (Fig. 4D). The PRC2 component, ASXL1, activates BAP-1 by increasing its affinity for ubiquitin (Sahtoe, van Dijk, Ekkebus, Ovaa, & Sixma, 2016). *ASXL1* mutations found in AML aberrantly enhance the DUB activity of BAP-1 and thus, deplete the levels of H3K27me[3] (Balasubramani et al., 2015). Such tumors mimic the effect of EZH2 inactivating mutations.

7. TARGETING DEREGULATED H3K27me

The convergence of many genetic aberrations in the deregulation of H3K27me in cancer has led to the development of inhibitors of the PRC2 complex catalytic core, EZH2. The first one identified, Deazaneplanocin A (DZNep) (Glazer et al., 1986), was shown to reactivate PRC2 target genes, lead to degradation of EZH2 and demonstrated antitumor activity

(Deb, Singh, & Gupta, 2014; Tan et al., 2007). DZNep inhibits SAH-hydrolase, a cofactor needed for the activity of many HMTs; therefore, it has a poor specificity toward EZH2. Hence, highly selective molecules directly targeting EZH2 were developed. These inhibitors directly compete for interaction with the methyl-group donor S-adenosyl methionine. They decrease levels of H3K27me$^{2/3}$ and reactivate transcription of PRC2/H3K27me^3 repressed genes involved in cell cycle regulation and differentiation (Beguelin et al., 2013; Kim, Bird, et al., 2013; Knutson et al., 2014; McCabe et al., 2012). Some studies have shown that these inhibitors have selective antitumor effects toward lymphoma cells harboring activating mutations in EZH2 (Beguelin et al., 2013). On the other hand, in GCB-type DLBCL, these inhibitors target equally WT and mutated EZH2 cells (Beguelin et al., 2013; McCabe et al., 2012). Elevated levels of H3K27me^3 and EZH2 expression do not correlate with the GOF mutations in EZH2 (Zhou et al., 2015), and cell sensitivity to EZH2 inhibitors does not always correlate with globally high levels of H3K27me^3. For instance, the over-expression of MMSET sensitizes MM cells to EZH2 inhibitors, even though genome-wide H3K27me^3 levels decrease. It appears that cancer cells showing increased H3K27me at tumor suppressing genes are more sensitive to EZH2i, as in the case of rhabdoid tumors lacking the SNF5 protein (Knutson et al., 2013).

Furthermore, loss of UTX in MM and T-ALL has been associated with increases in H3K27me^3 at specific loci, and correlates with increased sensitivity to EZH2i (Ezponda et al., 2014; Van der Meulen et al., 2015). Many cancers are negative for UTX (Ibragimova, Maradeo, Dulaimi, & Cairns, 2013; Nickerson et al., 2014), and therefore may benefit from therapy targeting EZH2.

Phase 1/2 clinical trials have been initiated using the EZH2 inhibitor tazemetostat (Epizyme), in patients with advanced solid tumors or with relapsed or refractory B-cell lymphoma. Tazemetostat demonstrates a favorable safety profile and tolerability. The overall response rate in B-cell lymphoma has reached 60%, where almost all responders were wild type for EZH2 (Nickerson et al., 2014; Ribrag et al., 2015) suggesting that EZH2 hyperactivity can be mimicked by other alterations. Interestingly, clinical activity was observed in patients with *INI1*-negative and *SMARCA4*-negative tumors, both leading to an inactive SWI/SNF complex, giving hope for patient with such tumors, which represent 20% of all cancers.

The status of chromatin regulators deregulated in cancer that cross talk with PRC2 should be taken into consideration while designing future

Potential markers for response to inhibitors of H3K27 methylation

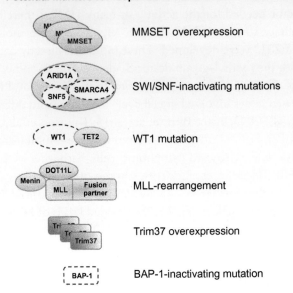

MMSET overexpression

SWI/SNF-inactivating mutations

WT1 mutation

MLL-rearrangement

Trim37 overexpression

BAP-1-inactivating mutation

Potential markers for response to inhibitors of H3K27 demethylation

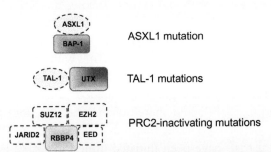

ASXL1 mutation

TAL-1 mutations

PRC2-inactivating mutations

Fig. 5 Many factors deregulated in cancer converge to increase or decrease H3K27me^3 in cancer, and they may represent new therapeutic targets, or biomarkers of response to existing agents. (See the color plate.)

clinical trials using drugs targeting H3K27 methylation (Fig. 5). It is yet to be proven whether the status of commonly deregulated chromatin enzymes could serve as biomarkers of response to EZH2i, such as *TRIM37* amplification in breast cancer, MMSET overexpression, the presence of MLL oncofusions, and *WT1*-inactivated tumors.

With any antitumor agent, there is the possibility that resistance will occur, and some studies have focused on modeling this phenomenon.

In an in vitro model of acquired resistance to EZH2i, secondary mutations where identified in wild-type and mutant EZH2 alleles (Gibaja et al., 2016). The presence of Ras pathway mutations, along with mutations in SWI/SNF, correlated with resistance to EZH2 inhibition (Baude, Lindroth, & Plass, 2014; De Raedt et al., 2011). These studies underlie the need to develop other EZH2 or PRC2 inhibitors and to design combination strategies.

EZH2 oncogenic activity has been attributed to nonenzymatic functions (Kim et al., 2015), and therefore inhibitors of its catalytic site may not fully suppress its tumor-promoting activity. Since the interaction of EED with EZH2 is essential for activity of the PRC2 complex (Cao et al., 2002; Chamberlain, Yee, & Magnuson, 2008; Denisenko et al., 1998; Han et al., 2007), a small molecule was developed to target the alpha-helical domain of EZH2 that binds EED and thus, disrupts this interaction (Kim, Bird, et al., 2013). This molecule, known as stabilized alpha-helix of EZH2 (SAH-EZH2) is specific to both EZH1 and 2, and leads to global dose-dependent decreases in H3K27me^3. SAH-EZH2 also leads to degradation of EZH2, eliminating both enzymatic and structural functions of EZH2. Notably, SAH-EZH2 is effective in some SWI/SNF-mutant cancers cell lines that rely on nonenzymatic functions of EZH2 and are resistant to catalytic EZH2 inhibitors. Moreover, an antiproliferative effect and induction of monocytic differentiation was observed upon treatment in leukemia cells harboring the AF9-MLL translocation or EZH2 activating mutations. SAH-EZH2 exhibits mechanistic differences with the first generation of catalytic inhibitors developed and therefore, the two synergize together to repress leukemic cells growth.

Approaches in epigenetic therapy have also recently focused on the development of molecules that block the "readers" of methyl mark, for instance the methyl mark on histone H4 lysine 20 (H4K20), which is involved in the DNA damage response, DNA replication, and mitotic condensation (James et al., 2013; Ma et al., 2014). Likewise, compounds targeting H3K27me "readers" may be developed to treat cancers showing a GOF of these factors. Recently, an inhibitor of CBX7 was identified and demonstrated interaction with key residues in the methyl-lysine binding pocket of CBX7 chromodomain (Ren et al., 2015). This molecule disrupts the interaction of CBX7 with H3K27me^3, and efficiently decreases its occupancy on INK4A/ARF locus in prostate cancer cells. However, no antitumor effect has been reported yet, and this drug exhibit poor specificity because it also targets several other CBX proteins.

Conversely, the PRC2 complex is inactivated in myeloid malignancies, for example T-ALL, and in peripheral nerve sheath tumors, where PRC2 inactivation correlates with loss of H3K27me^3 and activation of specific pathways. Elevated expression of the oncogenic transcription factor TAL-1 defines a major subgroup of T-ALL that has a specific expression signature (Ferrando et al., 2002). TAL-1 interacts with UTX to activate its target genes in these tumors (Benyoucef et al., 2016). An inhibitor of Jumonji H3K27 demethylase (Kruidenier et al., 2012) demonstrated antitumor activity in such tumors, which correlated with global increase in H3K27me and repression of the gene expression program specific to TAL-1 positive tumors (Ntziachristos et al., 2014). Jumonji H3K27 demethylase/UTX inhibitors may benefit patients presenting PRC2 inactivation.

In the same way, the H3K27M mutation in pediatric gliomas leads to decrease in H3K27me and these tumors demonstrate better susceptibility to inhibitors of the JmjD3 demethylase (Hashizume et al., 2014). Developing an epigenetic targeting strategy for tumors bearing K27M-H3.3 mutations seems complex, as these aberrations lead to both global decreases and local increases in H3K27me$^{2/3}$. Funato et al., who developed the pediatric glioma model discussed in Section 2, performed a chemical screen on their model using a commercially available small-molecule library of compounds that target epigenetic regulators (Funato et al., 2014). Their top hit was the menin inhibitor, MI-2. Menin is a component of MLL complexes, where it serves as a transcriptional cofactor. The Menin gene (*MEN1*) acts as a tumor suppressor in endocrine cancers (Matkar, Thiel, & Hua, 2013) but conversely, is highly oncogenic in MLL-rearranged leukemias (Yokoyama et al., 2005). Silencing of *MEN1* decreased proliferation specifically in H3.3K27M mutant cell lines and similarly, MI-2 also showed antineoplastic effects on cells derived from a patient sample.

Other therapeutic approaches may require the identification of biologically relevant transcription factors that normally compete with the PRC2 complex (such as NOTCH1 in T-ALL), or genes where H3K27me deregulation contributes to oncogenic transformation. The PRC2 complex has shown opposing functions in cancer; therefore, an appropriate use of EZH2/UTX inhibitors will need a careful consideration of the biological context, and certainly a better understanding of epigenetics regulation in different cancers. A more detailed mapping of these altered epigenomes is critical to ascertain which cancer subtypes could benefit from these drugs.

8. CONCLUSIONS AND FUTURE PERSPECTIVES

Alterations in levels and distribution of H3K27 methylation are a hallmark of transformation in many cancers and have been demonstrated to be a suitable target for antineoplastic therapy both in vitro and in vivo. Various epigenetic pathways work in concert to alter $H3K27me^3$ in cancer, thereby providing numerous approaches for targeting. The genes most affected by deregulated H3K27me are cancer-subtype-specific drivers of oncogenesis. Identification of the other transcription factors and epigenetic regulators also present at these affected genes may provide crucial insights for the design of new combination strategies and for the identification of biomarkers of response to those agents already being tested in the clinic, such as EZH2i. Many questions about how perturbations in H3K27me patterning leads to tumorigenesis remain, mostly due to conflicting reports of differences in the roles of the writers and readers of H3K27 methylation in different tissues, and even in different developmental stages. This highlights the need for more basic in vitro studies, mouse models, and careful validation of the drugs targeting this pathway in order to gain a more complete picture of the importance of this epigenetic mark.

ACKNOWLEDGMENTS

This work was supported by R01CA180475, a Leukemia and Lymphoma Society Specialized Center of Excellence grant (J.D.L.), CIHR operating Grant MOP-12863 (W.H.M.), and the Samuel Waxman Cancer Research Fund (J.D.L. and W.H.M.).

REFERENCES

Abdel-Wahab, O., Adli, M., LaFave, L. M., Gao, J., Hricik, T., Shih, A. H., et al. (2012). ASXL1 mutations promote myeloid transformation through loss of PRC2-mediated gene repression. *Cancer Cell, 22*, 180–193.

Adams, H., Fritzsche, F. R., Dirnhofer, S., Kristiansen, G., & Tzankov, A. (2010). Class I histone deacetylases 1, 2 and 3 are highly expressed in classical Hodgkin's lymphoma. *Expert Opinion on Therapeutic Targets, 14*, 577–584.

Agger, K., Cloos, P. A., Christensen, J., Pasini, D., Rose, S., Rappsilber, J., et al. (2007). UTX and JMJD3 are histone H3K27 demethylases involved in HOX gene regulation and development. *Nature, 449*, 731–734.

Ahmad, K., & Henikoff, S. (2002). The histone variant H3.3 marks active chromatin by replication-independent nucleosome assembly. *Molecular Cell, 9*, 1191–1200.

Asangani, I. A., Ateeq, B., Cao, Q., Dodson, L., Pandhi, M., Kunju, L. P., et al. (2013). Characterization of the EZH2-MMSET histone methyltransferase regulatory axis in cancer. *Molecular Cell, 49*, 80–93.

Bachmann, I. M., Halvorsen, O. J., Collett, K., Stefansson, I. M., Straume, O., Haukaas, S. A., et al. (2006). EZH2 expression is associated with high proliferation rate and aggressive tumor subgroups in cutaneous melanoma and cancers of the endometrium, prostate, and breast. *Journal of Clinical Oncology, 24*, 268–273.

Bailey, P., Chang, D. K., Nones, K., Johns, A. L., Patch, A. M., Gingras, M. C., et al. (2016). Genomic analyses identify molecular subtypes of pancreatic cancer. *Nature, 531*, 47–52.

Balasubramani, A., Larjo, A., Bassein, J. A., Chang, X., Hastie, R. B., Togher, S. M., et al. (2015). Cancer-associated ASXL1 mutations may act as gain-of-function mutations of the ASXL1-BAP1 complex. *Nature Communications, 6*, 7307.

Barsotti, A. M., Ryskin, M., Zhong, W., Zhang, W. G., Giannakou, A., Loreth, C., et al. (2015). Epigenetic reprogramming by tumor-derived EZH2 gain-of-function mutations promotes aggressive 3D cell morphologies and enhances melanoma tumor growth. *Oncotarget, 6*, 2928–2938.

Baude, A., Lindroth, A. M., & Plass, C. (2014). PRC2 loss amplifies Ras signaling in cancer. *Nature Genetics, 46*, 1154–1155.

Bea, S., Valdes-Mas, R., Navarro, A., Salaverria, I., Martin-Garcia, D., Jares, P., et al. (2013). Landscape of somatic mutations and clonal evolution in mantle cell lymphoma. *Proceedings of the National Academy of Sciences of the United States of America, 110*, 18250–18255.

Beguelin, W., Popovic, R., Teater, M., Jiang, Y., Bunting, K. L., Rosen, M., et al. (2013). EZH2 is required for germinal center formation and somatic EZH2 mutations promote lymphoid transformation. *Cancer Cell, 23*, 677–692.

Behjati, S., Tarpey, P. S., Presneau, N., Scheipl, S., Pillay, N., Van Loo, P., et al. (2013). Distinct H3F3A and H3F3B driver mutations define chondroblastoma and giant cell tumor of bone. *Nature Genetics, 45*, 1479–1482.

Behm, F. G., Raimondi, S. C., Frestedt, J. L., Liu, Q., Crist, W. M., Downing, J. R., et al. (1996). Rearrangement of the MLL gene confers a poor prognosis in childhood acute lymphoblastic leukemia, regardless of presenting age. *Blood, 87*, 2870–2877.

Bender, S., Tang, Y., Lindroth, A. M., Hovestadt, V., Jones, D. T., Kool, M., et al. (2013). Reduced H3K27me3 and DNA hypomethylation are major drivers of gene expression in K27M mutant pediatric high-grade gliomas. *Cancer Cell, 24*, 660–672.

Benyoucef, A., Palii, C. G., Wang, C., Porter, C. J., Chu, A., Dai, F., et al. (2016). UTX inhibition as selective epigenetic therapy against TAL1-driven T-cell acute lymphoblastic leukemia. *Genes & Development, 30*, 508–521.

Berdasco, M., & Esteller, M. (2013). Genetic syndromes caused by mutations in epigenetic genes. *Human Genetics, 132*, 359–383.

Bhatnagar, S., Gazin, C., Chamberlain, L., Ou, J., Zhu, X., Tushir, J. S., et al. (2014). TRIM37 is a new histone H2A ubiquitin ligase and breast cancer oncoprotein. *Nature, 516*, 116–120.

Bitler, B. G., Aird, K. M., Garipov, A., Li, H., Amatangelo, M., Kossenkov, A. V., et al. (2015). Synthetic lethality by targeting EZH2 methyltransferase activity in ARID1A-mutated cancers. *Nature Medicine, 21*, 231–238.

Blackledge, N. P., Farcas, A. M., Kondo, T., King, H. W., McGouran, J. F., Hanssen, L. L., et al. (2014). Variant PRC1 complex-dependent H2A ubiquitylation drives PRC2 recruitment and Polycomb domain formation. *Cell, 157*, 1445–1459.

Boulay, G., Rosnoblet, C., Guerardel, C., Angrand, P. O., & Leprince, D. (2011). Functional characterization of human Polycomb-like 3 isoforms identifies them as components of distinct EZH2 protein complexes. *The Biochemical Journal, 434*, 333–342.

Bracken, A. P., Pasini, D., Capra, M., Prosperini, E., Colli, E., & Helin, K. (2003). EZH2 is downstream of the pRB-E2F pathway, essential for proliferation and amplified in cancer. *The EMBO Journal, 22*, 5323–5335.

Brecqueville, M., Cervera, N., Adelaide, J., Rey, J., Carbuccia, N., Chaffanet, M., et al. (2011). Mutations and deletions of the SUZ12 Polycomb gene in myeloproliferative neoplasms. *Blood Cancer Journal, 1*, e33.

Brinkman, A. B., Gu, H., Bartels, S. J., Zhang, Y., Matarese, F., Simmer, F., et al. (2012). Sequential ChIP-bisulfite sequencing enables direct genome-scale investigation of chromatin and DNA methylation cross-talk. *Genome Research*, *22*, 1128–1138.

Brito, J. L., Walker, B., Jenner, M., Dickens, N. J., Brown, N. J., Ross, F. M., et al. (2009). MMSET deregulation affects cell cycle progression and adhesion regulons in t(4;14) myeloma plasma cells. *Haematologica*, *94*, 78–86.

Buczkowicz, P., Hoeman, C., Rakopoulos, P., Pajovic, S., Letourneau, L., Dzamba, M., et al. (2014). Genomic analysis of diffuse intrinsic pontine gliomas identifies three molecular subgroups and recurrent activating ACVR1 mutations. *Nature Genetics*, *46*, 451–456.

Bush, K. M., Yuen, B. T., Barrilleaux, B. L., Riggs, J. W., O'Geen, H., Cotterman, R. F., et al. (2013). Endogenous mammalian histone H3.3 exhibits chromatin-related functions during development. *Epigenetics & Chromatin*, *6*, 7.

Cao, R., Wang, L., Wang, H., Xia, L., Erdjument-Bromage, H., Tempst, P., et al. (2002). Role of histone H3 lysine 27 methylation in Polycomb-group silencing. *Science*, *298*, 1039–1043.

Cao, Q., Yu, J., Dhanasekaran, S. M., Kim, J. H., Mani, R. S., Tomlins, S. A., et al. (2008). Repression of E-cadherin by the polycomb group protein EZH2 in cancer. *Oncogene*, *27*, 7274–7284.

Cao, R., & Zhang, Y. (2004). The functions of E(Z)/EZH2-mediated methylation of lysine 27 in histone H3. *Current Opinion in Genetics & Development*, *14*, 155–164.

Carlotti, E., Wrench, D., Rosignoli, G., Marzec, J., Sangaralingam, A., Hazanov, L., et al. (2015). High throughput sequencing analysis of the immunoglobulin heavy chain gene from flow-sorted B cell sub-populations define the dynamics of follicular lymphoma clonal evolution. *PLoS One*, *10*, e0134833.

Cerami, E., Gao, J., Dogrusoz, U., Gross, B. E., Sumer, S. O., Aksoy, B. A., et al. (2012). The cBio cancer genomics portal: An open platform for exploring multidimensional cancer genomics data. *Cancer Discovery*, *2*, 401–404.

Chamberlain, S. J., Yee, D., & Magnuson, T. (2008). Polycomb repressive complex 2 is dispensable for maintenance of embryonic stem cell pluripotency. *Stem Cells*, *26*, 1496–1505.

Chan, K. M., Fang, D., Gan, H., Hashizume, R., Yu, C., Schroeder, M., et al. (2013). The histone H3.3K27M mutation in pediatric glioma reprograms H3K27 methylation and gene expression. *Genes & Development*, *27*, 985–990.

Chen, S., Yang, Z., Wilkinson, A. W., Deshpande, A. J., Sidoli, S., Krajewski, K., et al. (2015). The PZP domain of AF10 senses unmodified H3K27 to regulate DOT1L-mediated methylation of H3K79. *Molecular Cell*, *60*, 319–327.

Cho, Y. W., Hong, T., Hong, S., Guo, H., Yu, H., Kim, D., et al. (2007). PTIP associates with MLL3- and MLL4-containing histone H3 lysine 4 methyltransferase complex. *The Journal of Biological Chemistry*, *282*, 20395–20406.

Choi, J. H., Kwon, H. J., Yoon, B. I., Kim, J. H., Han, S. U., Joo, H. J., et al. (2001). Expression profile of histone deacetylase 1 in gastric cancer tissues. *Japanese Journal of Cancer Research: Gann*, *92*, 1300–1304.

Choi, H. J., Park, J. H., Park, M., Won, H. Y., Joo, H. S., Lee, C. H., et al. (2015). UTX inhibits EMT-induced breast CSC properties by epigenetic repression of EMT genes in cooperation with LSD1 and HDAC1. *EMBO Reports*, *16*, 1288–1298.

Czermin, B., Melfi, R., McCabe, D., Seitz, V., Imhof, A., & Pirrotta, V. (2002). Drosophila enhancer of Zeste/ESC complexes have a histone H3 methyltransferase activity that marks chromosomal Polycomb sites. *Cell*, *111*, 185–196.

De Raedt, T., Walton, Z., Yecies, J. L., Li, D., Chen, Y., Malone, C. F., et al. (2011). Exploiting cancer cell vulnerabilities to develop a combination therapy for Ras-driven tumors. *Cancer Cell*, *20*, 400–413.

Deb, G., Singh, A. K., & Gupta, S. (2014). EZH2: Not EZHY (easy) to deal. *Molecular Cancer Research, 12*, 639–653.

Delbarre, E., Jacobsen, B. M., Reiner, A. H., Sorensen, A. L., Kuntziger, T., & Collas, P. (2010). Chromatin environment of histone variant H3.3 revealed by quantitative imaging and genome-scale chromatin and DNA immunoprecipitation. *Molecular Biology of the Cell, 21*, 1872–1884.

Denisenko, O., Shnyreva, M., Suzuki, H., & Bomsztyk, K. (1998). Point mutations in the WD40 domain of Eed block its interaction with Ezh2. *Molecular and Cellular Biology, 18*, 5634–5642.

Deshpande, A. J., Deshpande, A., Sinha, A. U., Chen, L., Chang, J., Cihan, A., et al. (2014). AF10 regulates progressive H3K79 methylation and HOX gene expression in diverse AML subtypes. *Cancer Cell, 26*, 896–908.

Dey, A., Seshasayee, D., Noubade, R., French, D. M., Liu, J., Chaurushiya, M. S., et al. (2012). Loss of the tumor suppressor BAP1 causes myeloid transformation. *Science, 337*, 1541–1546.

Ene, C. I., Edwards, L., Riddick, G., Baysan, M., Woolard, K., Kotliarova, S., et al. (2012). Histone demethylase Jumonji D3 (JMJD3) as a tumor suppressor by regulating p53 protein nuclear stabilization. *PloS One, 7*, e51407.

Ernst, T., Chase, A. J., Score, J., Hidalgo-Curtis, C. E., Bryant, C., Jones, A. V., et al. (2010). Inactivating mutations of the histone methyltransferase gene EZH2 in myeloid disorders. *Nature Genetics, 42*, 722–726.

Ezponda, T., Popovic, R., Shah, M. Y., Martinez-Garcia, E., Zheng, Y., Min, D. J., et al. (2013). The histone methyltransferase MMSET/WHSC1 activates TWIST1 to promote an epithelial-mesenchymal transition and invasive properties of prostate cancer. *Oncogene, 32*, 2882–2890.

Ezponda, T., Popovic, R., Zheng, Y., Nabet, B., Will, C., Small, E. C., et al. (2014). *Loss of the histone demethylase UTX contributes to multiple myeloma and sensitizes cells to EZH2 inhibitors.* Paper presented at 56th annual meeting of the American-Society-of-Hematology (San Francisco, California).

Falkenberg, K. J., & Johnstone, R. W. (2014). Histone deacetylases and their inhibitors in cancer, neurological diseases and immune disorders. *Nature Reviews. Drug Discovery, 13*, 673–691.

Federico, A., Pallante, P., Bianco, M., Ferraro, A., Esposito, F., Monti, M., et al. (2009). Chromobox protein homologue 7 protein, with decreased expression in human carcinomas, positively regulates E-cadherin expression by interacting with the histone deacetylase 2 protein. *Cancer Research, 69*, 7079–7087.

Ferrando, A. A., Neuberg, D. S., Staunton, J., Loh, M. L., Huard, C., Raimondi, S. C., et al. (2002). Gene expression signatures define novel oncogenic pathways in T cell acute lymphoblastic leukemia. *Cancer Cell, 1*, 75–87.

Fiskus, W., Pranpat, M., Balasis, M., Herger, B., Rao, R., Chinnaiyan, A., et al. (2006). Histone deacetylase inhibitors deplete enhancer of zeste 2 and associated polycomb repressive complex 2 proteins in human acute leukemia cells. *Molecular Cancer Therapeutics, 5*, 3096–3104.

Fontebasso, A. M., Papillon-Cavanagh, S., Schwartzentruber, J., Nikbakht, H., Gerges, N., Fiset, P. O., et al. (2014). Recurrent somatic mutations in ACVR1 in pediatric midline high-grade astrocytoma. *Nature Genetics, 46*, 462–466.

Forzati, F., Federico, A., Pallante, P., Abbate, A., Esposito, F., Malapelle, U., et al. (2012). CBX7 is a tumor suppressor in mice and humans. *The Journal of Clinical Investigation, 122*, 612–623.

Friedman, J. M., Liang, G., Liu, C. C., Wolff, E. M., Tsai, Y. C., Ye, W., et al. (2009). The putative tumor suppressor microRNA-101 modulates the cancer epigenome by repressing the polycomb group protein EZH2. *Cancer Research, 69*, 2623–2629.

Funato, K., Major, T., Lewis, P. W., Allis, C. D., & Tabar, V. (2014). Use of human embryonic stem cells to model pediatric gliomas with H3.3K27M histone mutation. *Science*, *346*, 1529–1533.

Gannon, O. M., Merida de Long, L., Endo-Munoz, L., Hazar-Rethinam, M., & Saunders, N. A. (2013). Dysregulation of the repressive H3K27 trimethylation mark in head and neck squamous cell carcinoma contributes to dysregulated squamous differentiation. *Clinical Cancer Research*, *19*, 428–441.

Gao, J., Aksoy, B. A., Dogrusoz, U., Dresdner, G., Gross, B., Sumer, S. O., et al. (2013). Integrative analysis of complex cancer genomics and clinical profiles using the cBioPortal. *Science Signaling*, *6*, pl1.

Gibaja, V., Shen, F., Harari, J., Korn, J., Ruddy, D., Saenz-Vash, V., et al. (2016). Development of secondary mutations in wild-type and mutant EZH2 alleles cooperates to confer resistance to EZH2 inhibitors. *Oncogene*, *35*, 558–566.

Glazer, R. I., Hartman, K. D., Knode, M. C., Richard, M. M., Chiang, P. K., Tseng, C. K., et al. (1986). 3-Deazaneplanocin: A new and potent inhibitor of S-adenosylhomocysteine hydrolase and its effects on human promyelocytic leukemia cell line HL-60. *Biochemical and Biophysical Research Communications*, *135*, 688–694.

Goldberg, A. D., Banaszynski, L. A., Noh, K. M., Lewis, P. W., Elsaesser, S. J., Stadler, S., et al. (2010). Distinct factors control histone variant H3.3 localization at specific genomic regions. *Cell*, *140*, 678–691.

Grubach, L., Juhl-Christensen, C., Rethmeier, A., Olesen, L. H., Aggerholm, A., Hokland, P., et al. (2008). Gene expression profiling of Polycomb, Hox and Meis genes in patients with acute myeloid leukaemia. *European Journal of Haematology*, *81*, 112–122.

Gui, Y., Guo, G., Huang, Y., Hu, X., Tang, A., Gao, S., et al. (2011). Frequent mutations of chromatin remodeling genes in transitional cell carcinoma of the bladder. *Nature Genetics*, *43*, 875–878.

Guo, G., Sun, X., Chen, C., Wu, S., Huang, P., Li, Z., et al. (2013). Whole-genome and whole-exome sequencing of bladder cancer identifies frequent alterations in genes involved in sister chromatid cohesion and segregation. *Nature Genetics*, *45*, 1459–1463.

Han, Z., Xing, X., Hu, M., Zhang, Y., Liu, P., & Chai, J. (2007). Structural basis of EZH2 recognition by EED. *Structure*, *15*, 1306–1315.

Harbour, J. W., Onken, M. D., Roberson, E. D., Duan, S., Cao, L., Worley, L. A., et al. (2010). Frequent mutation of BAP1 in metastasizing uveal melanomas. *Science*, *330*, 1410–1413.

Hashizume, R., Andor, N., Ihara, Y., Lerner, R., Gan, H., Chen, X., et al. (2014). Pharmacologic inhibition of histone demethylation as a therapy for pediatric brainstem glioma. *Nature Medicine*, *20*, 1394–1396.

Ho, A. S., Kannan, K., Roy, D. M., Morris, L. G., Ganly, I., Katabi, N., et al. (2013). The mutational landscape of adenoid cystic carcinoma. *Nature Genetics*, *45*, 791–798.

Hodis, E., Watson, I. R., Kryukov, G. V., Arold, S. T., Imielinski, M., Theurillat, J. P., et al. (2012). A landscape of driver mutations in melanoma. *Cell*, *150*, 251–263.

Hong, S., Cho, Y. W., Yu, L. R., Yu, H., Veenstra, T. D., & Ge, K. (2007). Identification of JmjC domain-containing UTX and JMJD3 as histone H3 lysine 27 demethylases. *Proceedings of the National Academy of Sciences of the United States of America*, *104*, 18439–18444.

Ibragimova, I., Maradeo, M. E., Dulaimi, E., & Cairns, P. (2013). Aberrant promoter hypermethylation of PBRM1, BAP1, SETD2, KDM6A and other chromatin-modifying genes is absent or rare in clear cell RCC. *Epigenetics*, *8*, 486–493.

Inoue, D., Kitaura, J., Togami, K., Nishimura, K., Enomoto, Y., Uchida, T., et al. (2013). Myelodysplastic syndromes are induced by histone methylation-altering ASXL1 mutations. *The Journal of Clinical Investigation*, *123*, 4627–4640.

Issaeva, I., Zonis, Y., Rozovskaia, T., Orlovsky, K., Croce, C. M., Nakamura, T., et al. (2007). Knockdown of ALR (MLL2) reveals ALR target genes and leads to alterations in cell adhesion and growth. *Molecular and Cellular Biology, 27*, 1889–1903.

Jaffe, J. D., Wang, Y., Chan, H. M., Zhang, J., Huether, R., Kryukov, G. V., et al. (2013). Global chromatin profiling reveals NSD2 mutations in pediatric acute lymphoblastic leukemia. *Nature Genetics, 45*, 1386–1391.

James, L. I., Barsyte-Lovejoy, D., Zhong, N., Krichevsky, L., Korboukh, V. K., Herold, J. M., et al. (2013). Discovery of a chemical probe for the L3MBTL3 methyllysine reader domain. *Nature Chemical Biology, 9*, 184–191.

Jeon, Y., & Lee, J. T. (2011). YY1 tethers Xist RNA to the inactive X nucleation center. *Cell, 146*, 119–133.

Kalb, R., Latwiel, S., Baymaz, H. I., Jansen, P. W., Muller, C. W., Vermeulen, M., et al. (2014). Histone H2A monoubiquitination promotes histone H3 methylation in Polycomb repression. *Nature Structural & Molecular Biology, 21*, 569–571.

Kamminga, L. M., Bystrykh, L. V., de Boer, A., Houwer, S., Douma, J., Weersing, E., et al. (2006). The Polycomb group gene Ezh2 prevents hematopoietic stem cell exhaustion. *Blood, 107*, 2170–2179.

Karamitopoulou, E., Pallante, P., Zlobec, I., Tornillo, L., Carafa, V., Schaffner, T., et al. (2010). Loss of the CBX7 protein expression correlates with a more aggressive phenotype in pancreatic cancer. *European Journal of Cancer, 46*, 1438–1444.

Keats, J. J., Maxwell, C. A., Taylor, B. J., Hendzel, M. J., Chesi, M., Bergsagel, P. L., et al. (2005). Overexpression of transcripts originating from the MMSET locus characterizes all t(4;14)(p16;q32)-positive multiple myeloma patients. *Blood, 105*, 4060–4069.

Keats, J. J., Reiman, T., Maxwell, C. A., Taylor, B. J., Larratt, L. M., Mant, M. J., et al. (2003). In multiple myeloma, t(4;14)(p16;q32) is an adverse prognostic factor irrespective of FGFR3 expression. *Blood, 101*, 1520–1529.

Khan, S. N., Jankowska, A. M., Mahfouz, R., Dunbar, A. J., Sugimoto, Y., Hosono, N., et al. (2013). Multiple mechanisms deregulate EZH2 and histone H3 lysine 27 epigenetic changes in myeloid malignancies. *Leukemia, 27*, 1301–1309.

Khuong-Quang, D. A., Buczkowicz, P., Rakopoulos, P., Liu, X. Y., Fontebasso, A. M., Bouffet, E., et al. (2012). K27M mutation in histone H3.3 defines clinically and biologically distinct subgroups of pediatric diffuse intrinsic pontine gliomas. *Acta Neuropathologica, 124*, 439–447.

Kia, S. K., Gorski, M. M., Giannakopoulos, S., & Verrijzer, C. P. (2008). SWI/SNF mediates polycomb eviction and epigenetic reprogramming of the INK4b-ARF-INK4a locus. *Molecular and Cellular Biology, 28*, 3457–3464.

Kim, W., Bird, G. H., Neff, T., Guo, G., Kerenyi, M. A., Walensky, L. D., et al. (2013). Targeted disruption of the EZH2-EED complex inhibits EZH2-dependent cancer. *Nature Chemical Biology, 9*, 643–650.

Kim, H., Kang, K., & Kim, J. (2009). AEBP2 as a potential targeting protein for polycomb repression complex PRC2. *Nucleic Acids Research, 37*, 2940–2950.

Kim, K. H., Kim, W., Howard, T. P., Vazquez, F., Tsherniak, A., Wu, J. N., et al. (2015). SWI/SNF-mutant cancers depend on catalytic and non-catalytic activity of EZH2. *Nature Medicine, 21*, 1491–1496.

Kim, E., Kim, M., Woo, D. H., Shin, Y., Shin, J., Chang, N., et al. (2013). Phosphorylation of EZH2 activates STAT3 signaling via STAT3 methylation and promotes tumorigenicity of glioblastoma stem-like cells. *Cancer Cell, 23*, 839–852.

Kim, J. H., Sharma, A., Dhar, S. S., Lee, S. H., Gu, B., Chan, C. H., et al. (2014). UTX and MLL4 coordinately regulate transcriptional programs for cell proliferation and invasiveness in breast cancer cells. *Cancer Research, 74*, 1705–1717.

Kim, J., & Yu, J. (2012). Interrogating genomic and epigenomic data to understand prostate cancer. *Biochimica et Biophysica Acta, 1825*, 186–196.

Klauke, K., Radulovic, V., Broekhuis, M., Weersing, E., Zwart, E., Olthof, S., et al. (2013). Polycomb Cbx family members mediate the balance between haematopoietic stem cell self-renewal and differentiation. *Nature Cell Biology*, *15*, 353–362.

Kleer, C. G., Cao, Q., Varambally, S., Shen, R., Ota, I., Tomlins, S. A., et al. (2003). EZH2 is a marker of aggressive breast cancer and promotes neoplastic transformation of breast epithelial cells. *Proceedings of the National Academy of Sciences of the United States of America*, *100*, 11606–11611.

Knutson, S. K., Kawano, S., Minoshima, Y., Warholic, N. M., Huang, K. C., Xiao, Y., et al. (2014). Selective inhibition of EZH2 by EPZ-6438 leads to potent antitumor activity in EZH2 mutant non-Hodgkin lymphoma. *Molecular Cancer Therapeutics*, *13*(4), 842–854.

Knutson, S. K., Warholic, N. M., Wigle, T. J., Klaus, C. R., Allain, C. J., Raimondi, A., et al. (2013). Durable tumor regression in genetically altered malignant rhabdoid tumors by inhibition of methyltransferase EZH2. *Proceedings of the National Academy of Sciences of the United States of America*, *110*, 7922–7927.

Kong, D., Heath, E., Chen, W., Cher, M. L., Powell, I., Heilbrun, L., et al. (2012). Loss of let-7 up-regulates EZH2 in prostate cancer consistent with the acquisition of cancer stem cell signatures that are attenuated by BR-DIM. *PloS One*, *7*, e33729.

Kouzarides, T. (2007). Chromatin modifications and their function. *Cell*, *128*, 693–705.

Kruidenier, L., Chung, C. W., Cheng, Z., Liddle, J., Che, K., Joberty, G., et al. (2012). A selective jumonji H3K27 demethylase inhibitor modulates the proinflammatory macrophage response. *Nature*, *488*, 404–408.

Kuo, A. J., Cheung, P., Chen, K., Zee, B. M., Kioi, M., Lauring, J., et al. (2011). NSD2 links dimethylation of histone H3 at lysine 36 to oncogenic programming. *Molecular Cell*, *44*, 609–620.

Kuzmuchev, A., Nishioka, K., Erdjument-Bromage, H., Tempst, P., & Reinberg, D. (2002). Histone methyltransferase activity associated with a human multiprotein complex containing the Enhancer of Zeste protein. *Genes and Development*, *16*, 2893–2905.

LaFave, L. M., Beguelin, W., Koche, R., Teater, M., Spitzer, B., Chramiec, A., et al. (2015). Loss of BAP1 function leads to EZH2-dependent transformation. *Nature Medicine*, *21*, 1344–1349.

Lauring, J., Abukhdeir, A. M., Konishi, H., Garay, J. P., Gustin, J. P., Wang, Q., et al. (2008). The multiple myeloma associated MMSET gene contributes to cellular adhesion, clonogenic growth, and tumorigenicity. *Blood*, *111*, 856–864.

Lawrence, M. S., Stojanov, P., Mermel, C. H., Robinson, J. T., Garraway, L. A., Golub, T. R., et al. (2014). Discovery and saturation analysis of cancer genes across 21 tumour types. *Nature*, *505*, 495–501.

Lee, W., Teckie, S., Wiesner, T., Ran, L., Prieto Granada, C. N., Lin, M., et al. (2014). PRC2 is recurrently inactivated through EED or SUZ12 loss in malignant peripheral nerve sheath tumors. *Nature Genetics*, *46*, 1227–1232.

Lee, M. G., Villa, R., Trojer, P., Norman, J., Yan, K. P., Reinberg, D., et al. (2007). Demethylation of H3K27 regulates polycomb recruitment and H2A ubiquitination. *Science*, *318*, 447–450.

Lewis, P. W., Elsaesser, S. J., Noh, K. M., Stadler, S. C., & Allis, C. D. (2010). Daxx is an H3.3-specific histone chaperone and cooperates with ATRX in replication-independent chromatin assembly at telomeres. *Proceedings of the National Academy of Sciences of the United States of America*, *107*, 14075–14080.

Lewis, P. W., Muller, M. M., Koletsky, M. S., Cordero, F., Lin, S., Banaszynski, L. A., et al. (2013). Inhibition of PRC2 activity by a gain-of-function H3 mutation found in pediatric glioblastoma. *Science*, *340*, 857–861.

Li, X., Isono, K., Yamada, D., Endo, T. A., Endoh, M., Shinga, J., et al. (2011). Mammalian polycomb-like Pcl2/Mtf2 is a novel regulatory component of PRC2 that can differentially modulate polycomb activity both at the Hox gene cluster and at Cdkn2a genes. *Molecular and Cellular Biology, 31*, 351–364.

Li, G., Margueron, R., Ku, M., Chambon, P., Bernstein, B. E., & Reinberg, D. (2010). Jarid2 and PRC2, partners in regulating gene expression. *Genes & Development, 24*, 368–380.

Lin, C. J., Conti, M., & Ramalho-Santos, M. (2013). Histone variant H3.3 maintains a decondensed chromatin state essential for mouse preimplantation development. *Development, 140*, 3624–3634.

Ma, A., Yu, W., Li, F., Bleich, R. M., Herold, J. M., Butler, K. V., et al. (2014). Discovery of a selective, substrate-competitive inhibitor of the lysine methyltransferase SETD8. *Journal of Medicinal Chemistry, 57*, 6822–6833.

Majer, C. R., Jin, L., Scott, M. P., Knutson, S. K., Kuntz, K. W., Keilhack, H., et al. (2012). A687V EZH2 is a gain-of-function mutation found in lymphoma patients. *FEBS Letters, 586*, 3448–3451.

Margueron, R., Justin, N., Ohno, K., Sharpe, M. L., Son, J., Drury, W. J., 3rd, et al. (2009). Role of the polycomb protein EED in the propagation of repressive histone marks. *Nature, 461*, 762–767.

Margueron, R., Li, G., Sarma, K., Blais, A., Zavadil, J., Woodcock, C. L., et al. (2008). Ezh1 and Ezh2 maintain repressive chromatin through different mechanisms. *Molecular Cell, 32*, 503–518.

Marquard, L., Gjerdrum, L. M., Christensen, I. J., Jensen, P. B., Sehested, M., & Ralfkiaer, E. (2008). Prognostic significance of the therapeutic targets histone deacetylase 1, 2, 6 and acetylated histone H4 in cutaneous T-cell lymphoma. *Histopathology, 53*, 267–277.

Martinez-Garcia, E., Popovic, R., Min, D. J., Sweet, S. M., Thomas, P. M., Zamdborg, L., et al. (2011). The MMSET histone methyl transferase switches global histone methylation and alters gene expression in t(4;14) multiple myeloma cells. *Blood, 117*, 211–220.

Matkar, S., Thiel, A., & Hua, X. (2013). Menin: A scaffold protein that controls gene expression and cell signaling. *Trends in Biochemical Sciences, 38*, 394–402.

McCabe, M. T., Graves, A. P., Ganji, G., Diaz, E., Halsey, W. S., Jiang, Y., et al. (2012). Mutation of A677 in histone methyltransferase EZH2 in human B-cell lymphoma promotes hypertrimethylation of histone H3 on lysine 27 (H3K27). *Proceedings of the National Academy of Sciences of the United States of America, 109*, 2989–2994.

Monti, S., Chapuy, B., Takeyama, K., Rodig, S. J., Hao, Y., Yeda, K. T., et al. (2012). Integrative analysis reveals an outcome-associated and targetable pattern of p53 and cell cycle deregulation in diffuse large B cell lymphoma. *Cancer Cell, 22*, 359–372.

Morin, R. D., Johnson, N. A., Severson, T. M., Mungall, A. J., An, J., Goya, R., et al. (2010). Somatic mutations altering EZH2 (Tyr641) in follicular and diffuse large B-cell lymphomas of germinal-center origin. *Nature Genetics, 42*, 181–185.

Muller, J., Hart, C. M., Francis, N. J., Vargas, M. L., Sengupta, A., Wild, B., et al. (2002). Histone methyltransferase activity of a *Drosophila* Polycomb group repressor complex. *Cell, 111*, 197–208.

Mulligan, P., Westbrook, T. F., Ottinger, M., Pavlova, N., Chang, B., Macia, E., et al. (2008). CDYL bridges REST and histone methyltransferases for gene repression and suppression of cellular transformation. *Molecular Cell, 32*, 718–726.

Neff, T., Sinha, A. U., Kluk, M. J., Zhu, N., Khattab, M. H., Stein, L., et al. (2012). Polycomb repressive complex 2 is required for MLL-AF9 leukemia. *Proceedings of the National Academy of Sciences of the United States of America, 109*, 5028–5033.

Nekrasov, M., Klymenko, T., Fraterman, S., Papp, B., Oktaba, K., Kocher, T., et al. (2007). Pcl-PRC2 is needed to generate high levels of H3-K27 trimethylation at Polycomb target genes. *The EMBO Journal, 26*, 4078–4088.

Ng, S. B., Selvarajan, V., Huang, G., Zhou, J., Feldman, A. L., Law, M., et al. (2011). Activated oncogenic pathways and therapeutic targets in extranodal nasal-type NK/T cell lymphoma revealed by gene expression profiling. *The Journal of Pathology, 223*, 496–510.

Nickerson, M. L., Dancik, G. M., Im, K. M., Edwards, M. G., Turan, S., Brown, J., et al. (2014). Concurrent alterations in TERT, KDM6A, and the BRCA pathway in bladder cancer. *Clinical Cancer Research, 20,* 4935–4948.

Nikoloski, G., Langemeijer, S. M., Kuiper, R. P., Knops, R., Massop, M., Tonnissen, E. R., et al. (2010). Somatic mutations of the histone methyltransferase gene EZH2 in myelodysplastic syndromes. *Nature Genetics, 42,* 665–667.

Ntziachristos, P., Tsirigos, A., Van Vlierberghe, P., Nedjic, J., Trimarchi, T., Flaherty, M. S., et al. (2012). Genetic inactivation of the polycomb repressive complex 2 in T cell acute lymphoblastic leukemia. *Nature Medicine, 18,* 298–301.

Ntziachristos, P., Tsirigos, A., Welstead, G. G., Trimarchi, T., Bakogianni, S., Xu, L., et al. (2014). Contrasting roles of histone 3 lysine 27 demethylases in acute lymphoblastic leukaemia. *Nature, 514,* 513–517.

Oyer, J. A., Huang, X., Zheng, Y., Shim, J., Ezponda, T., Carpenter, Z., et al. (2014). Point mutation E1099K in MMSET/NSD2 enhances its methyltranferase activity and leads to altered global chromatin methylation in lymphoid malignancies. *Leukemia, 28,* 198–201.

Pallante, P., Sepe, R., Federico, A., Forzati, F., Bianco, M., & Fusco, A. (2014). CBX7 modulates the expression of genes critical for cancer progression. *PloS One, 9,* e98295.

Pasini, D., Bracken, A. P., Hansen, J. B., Capillo, M., & Helin, K. (2007). The polycomb group protein Suz12 is required for embryonic stem cell differentiation. *Molecular and Cellular Biology, 27,* 3769–3779.

Pasini, D., Bracken, A. P., Jensen, M. R., Lazzerini Denchi, E., & Helin, K. (2004). Suz12 is essential for mouse development and for EZH2 histone methyltransferase activity. *The EMBO Journal, 23,* 4061–4071.

Pasini, D., Cloos, P. A., Walfridsson, J., Olsson, L., Bukowski, J. P., Johansen, J. V., et al. (2010). JARID2 regulates binding of the Polycomb repressive complex 2 to target genes in ES cells. *Nature, 464,* 306–310.

Pasini, D., Malatesta, M., Jung, H. R., Walfridsson, J., Willer, A., Olsson, L., et al. (2010). Characterization of an antagonistic switch between histone H3 lysine 27 methylation and acetylation in the transcriptional regulation of Polycomb group target genes. *Nucleic Acids Research, 38,* 4958–4969.

Pasqualucci, L., Dominguez-Sola, D., Chiarenza, A., Fabbri, G., Grunn, A., Trifonov, V., et al. (2011). Inactivating mutations of acetyltransferase genes in B-cell lymphoma. *Nature, 471,* 189–195.

Pena-Llopis, S., Vega-Rubin-de-Celis, S., Liao, A., Leng, N., Pavia-Jimenez, A., Wang, S., et al. (2012). BAP1 loss defines a new class of renal cell carcinoma. *Nature Genetics, 44,* 751–759.

Peng, J. C., Valouev, A., Swigut, T., Zhang, J., Zhao, Y., Sidow, A., et al. (2009). Jarid2/Jumonji coordinates control of PRC2 enzymatic activity and target gene occupancy in pluripotent cells. *Cell, 139,* 1290–1302.

Popovic, R., Martinez, E., Zhang, Q., Ezponda, T., Jiang, Y., Shah, M. Y., et al. (2012). MMSET dysregulates gene expression in myeloma through global and focal changes in H3K36 and H3K27 methylation. *ASH Annual Meeting Abstracts, 120,* 523.

Rabello Ddo, A., Lucena-Araujo, A. R., Alves-Silva, J. C., da Eira, V. B., de Vasconcellos, M. C., de Oliveira, F. M., et al. (2015). Overexpression of EZH2 associates with a poor prognosis in chronic lymphocytic leukemia. *Blood Cells, Molecules & Diseases, 54,* 97–102.

Rampal, R., Alkalin, A., Madzo, J., Vasanthakumar, A., Pronier, E., Patel, J., et al. (2014). DNA hydroxymethylation profiling reveals that WT1 mutations result in loss of TET2 function in acute myeloid leukemia. *Cell Reports, 9,* 1841–1855.

Ray-Gallet, D., Quivy, J. P., Scamps, C., Martini, E. M., Lipinski, M., & Almouzni, G. (2002). HIRA is critical for a nucleosome assembly pathway independent of DNA synthesis. *Molecular Cell, 9,* 1091–1100.

Ren, C., Morohashi, K., Plotnikov, A. N., Jakoncic, J., Smith, S. G., Li, J., et al. (2015). Small-molecule modulators of methyl-lysine binding for the CBX7 chromodomain. *Chemistry & Biology*, *22*, 161–168.

Ribrag, V., Soria, J.-C., Michot, J.-M., Schmitt, A., Postel-Vinay, S., Bijou, F., et al. (2015). *Phase 1 study of tazemetostat (EPZ-6438), an inhibitor of enhancer of zeste-homolog 2 (EZH2): Preliminary safety and activity in relapsed or refractory non-Hodgkin lymphoma (NHL) patients.* Paper presented at: 57th Annual Meeting of the American-Society-of-Hematology (Orlando, Florida).

Sahtoe, D. D., van Dijk, W. J., Ekkebus, R., Ovaa, H., & Sixma, T. K. (2016). BAP1/ASXL1 recruitment and activation for H2A deubiquitination. *Nature Communications*, *7*, 10292.

Saramaki, O. R., Tammela, T. L., Martikainen, P. M., Vessella, R. L., & Visakorpi, T. (2006). The gene for polycomb group protein enhancer of zeste homolog 2 (EZH2) is amplified in late-stage prostate cancer. *Genes, Chromosomes & Cancer*, *45*, 639–645.

Sasaki, M., Yamaguchi, J., Itatsu, K., Ikeda, H., & Nakanuma, Y. (2008). Over-expression of polycomb group protein EZH2 relates to decreased expression of p16 INK4a in cholangiocarcinogenesis in hepatolithiasis. *The Journal of Pathology*, *215*, 175–183.

Sashida, G., Harada, H., Matsui, H., Oshima, M., Yui, M., Harada, Y., et al. (2014). Ezh2 loss promotes development of myelodysplastic syndrome but attenuates its predisposition to leukaemic transformation. *Nature Communications*, *5*, 4177.

Schuettengruber, B., Martinez, A. M., Iovino, N., & Cavalli, G. (2011). Trithorax group proteins: Switching genes on and keeping them active. *Nature Reviews Molecular Cell Biology*, *12*, 799–814.

Schwartzentruber, J., Korshunov, A., Liu, X. Y., Jones, D. T., Pfaff, E., Jacob, K., et al. (2012). Driver mutations in histone H3.3 and chromatin remodelling genes in paediatric glioblastoma. *Nature*, *482*, 226–231.

Score, J., Hidalgo-Curtis, C., Jones, A. V., Winkelmann, N., Skinner, A., Ward, D., et al. (2012). Inactivation of polycomb repressive complex 2 components in myeloproliferative and myelodysplastic/myeloproliferative neoplasms. *Blood*, *119*, 1208–1213.

Shi, J., Wang, E., Zuber, J., Rappaport, A., Taylor, M., Johns, C., et al. (2013). The Polycomb complex PRC2 supports aberrant self-renewal in a mouse model of MLL-AF9;Nras(G12D) acute myeloid leukemia. *Oncogene*, *32*, 930–938.

Simon, C., Chagraoui, J., Krosl, J., Gendron, P., Wilhelm, B., Lemieux, S., et al. (2012). A key role for EZH2 and associated genes in mouse and human adult T-cell acute leukemia. *Genes & Development*, *26*, 651–656.

Sinha, S., Thomas, D., Yu, L., Gentles, A. J., Jung, N., Corces-Zimmerman, M. R., et al. (2015). Mutant WT1 is associated with DNA hypermethylation of PRC2 targets in AML and responds to EZH2 inhibition. *Blood*, *125*, 316–326.

Sneeringer, C. J., Scott, M. P., Kuntz, K. W., Knutson, S. K., Pollock, R. M., Richon, V. M., et al. (2010). Coordinated activities of wild-type plus mutant EZH2 drive tumor-associated hypertrimethylation of lysine 27 on histone H3 (H3K27) in human B-cell lymphomas. *Proceedings of the National Academy of Sciences of the United States of America*, *107*, 20980–20985.

Song, C., Pan, X., Ge, Z., Gowda, C., Ding, Y., Li, H., et al. (2015). Epigenetic regulation of gene expression by Ikaros, HDAC1 and Casein Kinase II in leukemia. *Leukemia*.

Statham, A. L., Robinson, M. D., Song, J. Z., Coolen, M. W., Stirzaker, C., & Clark, S. J. (2012). Bisulfite sequencing of chromatin immunoprecipitated DNA (BisChIP-seq) directly informs methylation status of histone-modified DNA. *Genome Research*, *22*, 1120–1127.

Stransky, N., Egloff, A. M., Tward, A. D., Kostic, A. D., Cibulskis, K., Sivachenko, A., et al. (2011). The mutational landscape of head and neck squamous cell carcinoma. *Science*, *333*, 1157–1160.

Sturm, D., Witt, H., Hovestadt, V., Khuong-Quang, D. A., Jones, D. T., Konermann, C., et al. (2012). Hotspot mutations in H3F3A and IDH1 define distinct epigenetic and biological subgroups of glioblastoma. *Cancer Cell, 22*, 425–437.

Szenker, E., Ray-Gallet, D., & Almouzni, G. (2011). The double face of the histone variant H3.3. *Cell Research, 21*, 421–434.

Tan, J., Yang, X., Zhuang, L., Jiang, X., Chen, W., Lee, P. L., et al. (2007). Pharmacologic disruption of Polycomb-repressive complex 2-mediated gene repression selectively induces apoptosis in cancer cells. *Genes & Development, 21*, 1050–1063.

Tanaka, S., Miyagi, S., Sashida, G., Chiba, T., Yuan, J., Mochizuki-Kashio, M., et al. (2012). Ezh2 augments leukemogenicity by reinforcing differentiation blockage in acute myeloid leukemia. *Blood, 120*, 1107–1117.

Testa, J. R., Cheung, M., Pei, J., Below, J. E., Tan, Y., Sementino, E., et al. (2011). Germline BAP1 mutations predispose to malignant mesothelioma. *Nature Genetics, 43*, 1022–1025.

Tie, F., Banerjee, R., Conrad, P. A., Scacheri, P. C., & Harte, P. J. (2012). Histone demethylase UTX and chromatin remodeler BRM bind directly to CBP and modulate acetylation of histone H3 lysine 27. *Molecular and Cellular Biology, 32*, 2323–2334.

Tie, F., Banerjee, R., Stratton, C. A., Prasad-Sinha, J., Stepanik, V., Zlobin, A., et al. (2009). CBP-mediated acetylation of histone H3 lysine 27 antagonizes Drosophila Polycomb silencing. *Development, 136*, 3131–3141.

Ueda, T., Sanada, M., Matsui, H., Yamasaki, N., Honda, Z. I., Shih, L. Y., et al. (2012). EED mutants impair polycomb repressive complex 2 in myelodysplastic syndrome and related neoplasms. *Leukemia, 26*, 2557–2560.

Van der Meulen, J., Sanghvi, V., Mavrakis, K., Durinck, K., Fang, F., Matthijssens, F., et al. (2015). The H3K27me3 demethylase UTX is a gender-specific tumor suppressor in T-cell acute lymphoblastic leukemia. *Blood, 125*, 13–21.

van der Vlag, J., & Otte, A. P. (1999). Transcriptional repression mediated by the human polycomb-group protein EED involves histone deacetylation. *Nature Genetics, 23*, 474–478.

van Haaften, G., Dalgliesh, G. L., Davies, H., Chen, L., Bignell, G., Greenman, C., et al. (2009). Somatic mutations of the histone H3K27 demethylase gene UTX in human cancer. *Nature Genetics, 41*, 521–523.

Varambally, S., Cao, Q., Mani, R. S., Shankar, S., Wang, X., Ateeq, B., et al. (2008). Genomic loss of microRNA-101 leads to overexpression of histone methyltransferase EZH2 in cancer. *Science, 322*, 1695–1699.

Varambally, S., Dhanasekaran, S. M., Zhou, M., Barrette, T. R., Kumar-Sinha, C., Sanda, M. G., et al. (2002). The polycomb group protein EZH2 is involved in progression of prostate cancer. *Nature, 419*, 624–629.

Wada, T., Kikuchi, J., Nishimura, N., Shimizu, R., Kitamura, T., & Furukawa, Y. (2009). Expression levels of histone deacetylases determine the cell fate of hematopoietic progenitors. *The Journal of Biological Chemistry, 284*, 30673–30683.

Waddell, N., Pajic, M., Patch, A. M., Chang, D. K., Kassahn, K. S., Bailey, P., et al. (2015). Whole genomes redefine the mutational landscape of pancreatic cancer. *Nature, 518*, 495–501.

Walker, E., Chang, W. Y., Hunkapiller, J., Cagney, G., Garcha, K., Torchia, J., et al. (2010). Polycomb-like 2 associates with PRC2 and regulates transcriptional networks during mouse embryonic stem cell self-renewal and differentiation. *Cell Stem Cell, 6*, 153–166.

Wang, G. G., Cai, L., Pasillas, M. P., & Kamps, M. P. (2007). NUP98-NSD1 links H3K36 methylation to Hox-A gene activation and leukaemogenesis. *Nature Cell Biology, 9*, 804–812.

Wang, X., Dai, H., Wang, Q., Wang, Q., Xu, Y., Wang, Y., et al. (2013). EZH2 mutations are related to low blast percentage in bone marrow and -7/del(7q) in de novo acute myeloid leukemia. *PloS One*, *8*, e61341.

Wang, C., Liu, Z., Woo, C. W., Li, Z., Wang, L., Wei, J. S., et al. (2012). EZH2 mediates epigenetic silencing of neuroblastoma suppressor genes CASZ1, CLU, RUNX3, and NGFR. *Cancer Research*, *72*, 315–324.

Wang, G. G., Song, J., Wang, Z., Dormann, H. L., Casadio, F., Li, H., et al. (2009). Haematopoietic malignancies caused by dysregulation of a chromatin-binding PHD finger. *Nature*, *459*, 847–851.

Wang, Y., Xiao, M., Chen, X., Chen, L., Xu, Y., Lv, L., et al. (2015). WT1 recruits TET2 to regulate its target gene expression and suppress leukemia cell proliferation. *Molecular Cell*, *57*, 662–673.

Wiedemann, S. M., Mildner, S. N., Bonisch, C., Israel, L., Maiser, A., Matheisl, S., et al. (2010). Identification and characterization of two novel primate-specific histone H3 variants, H3.X and H3.Y. *The Journal of Cell Biology*, *190*, 777–791.

Wilson, B. G., Wang, X., Shen, X., McKenna, E. S., Lemieux, M. E., Cho, Y. J., et al. (2010). Epigenetic antagonism between polycomb and SWI/SNF complexes during oncogenic transformation. *Cancer Cell*, *18*, 316–328.

Witt, O., Albig, W., & Doenecke, D. (1996). Testis-specific expression of a novel human H3 histone gene. *Experimental Cell Research*, *229*, 301–306.

Wu, G., Broniscer, A., McEachron, T. A., Lu, C., Paugh, B. S., Becksfort, J., et al. (2012). Somatic histone H3 alterations in pediatric diffuse intrinsic pontine gliomas and nonbrainstem glioblastomas. *Nature Genetics*, *44*, 251–253.

Wu, X., Northcott, P. A., Dubuc, A., Dupuy, A. J., Shih, D. J., Witt, H., et al. (2012). Clonal selection drives genetic divergence of metastatic medulloblastoma. *Nature*, *482*, 529–533.

Xu, C., Bian, C., Yang, W., Galka, M., Ouyang, H., Chen, C., et al. (2010). Binding of different histone marks differentially regulates the activity and specificity of polycomb repressive complex 2 (PRC2). *Proceedings of the National Academy of Sciences of the United States of America*, *107*, 19266–19271.

Xu, F., Li, X., Wu, L., Zhang, Q., Yang, R., Yang, Y., et al. (2011). Overexpression of the EZH2, RING1 and BMI1 genes is common in myelodysplastic syndromes: Relation to adverse epigenetic alteration and poor prognostic scoring. *Annals of Hematology*, *90*, 643–653.

Xu, B., On, D. M., Ma, A., Parton, T., Konze, K. D., Pattenden, S. G., et al. (2015). Selective inhibition of EZH2 and EZH1 enzymatic activity by a small molecule suppresses MLL-rearranged leukemia. *Blood*, *125*, 346–357.

Xu, K., Wu, Z. J., Groner, A. C., He, H. H., Cai, C., Lis, R. T., et al. (2012). EZH2 oncogenic activity in castration-resistant prostate cancer cells is Polycomb-independent. *Science*, *338*, 1465–1469.

Yan, J., Ng, S. B., Tay, J. L., Lin, B., Koh, T. L., Tan, J., et al. (2013). EZH2 overexpression in natural killer/T-cell lymphoma confers growth advantage independently of histone methyltransferase activity. *Blood*, *121*, 4512–4520.

Yap, D. B., Chu, J., Berg, T., Schapira, M., Cheng, S. W., Moradian, A., et al. (2011). Somatic mutations at EZH2 Y641 act dominantly through a mechanism of selectively altered PRC2 catalytic activity, to increase H3K27 trimethylation. *Blood*, *117*, 2451–2459.

Yokoyama, A., Somervaille, T. C., Smith, K. S., Rozenblatt-Rosen, O., Meyerson, M., & Cleary, M. L. (2005). The menin tumor suppressor protein is an essential oncogenic cofactor for MLL-associated leukemogenesis. *Cell*, *123*, 207–218.

Yuan, W., Wu, T., Fu, H., Dai, C., Wu, H., Liu, N., et al. (2012). Dense chromatin activates Polycomb repressive complex 2 to regulate H3 lysine 27 methylation. *Science*, *337*, 971–975.

Yuan, W., Xu, M., Huang, C., Liu, N., Chen, S., & Zhu, B. (2011). H3K36 methylation antagonizes PRC2-mediated H3K27 methylation. *The Journal of Biological Chemistry*, *286*, 7983–7989.

Zhang, J., Ding, L., Holmfeldt, L., Wu, G., Heatley, S. L., Payne-Turner, D., et al. (2012). The genetic basis of early T-cell precursor acute lymphoblastic leukaemia. *Nature*, *481*, 157–163.

Zhang, Z., Jones, A., Sun, C. W., Li, C., Chang, C. W., Joo, H. Y., et al. (2011). PRC2 complexes with JARID2, MTF2, and esPRC2p48 in ES cells to modulate ES cell pluripotency and somatic cell reprogramming. *Stem Cells*, *29*, 229–240.

Zhang, Z., Yamashita, H., Toyama, T., Sugiura, H., Ando, Y., Mita, K., et al. (2005). Quantitation of HDAC1 mRNA expression in invasive carcinoma of the breast. *Breast Cancer Research and Treatment*, *94*, 11–16.

Zhang, Y., Yang, X., Gui, B., Xie, G., Zhang, D., Shang, Y., et al. (2011). Corepressor protein CDYL functions as a molecular bridge between polycomb repressor complex 2 and repressive chromatin mark trimethylated histone lysine 27. *The Journal of Biological Chemistry*, *286*, 42414–42425.

Zhao, J., Ohsumi, T. K., Kung, J. T., Ogawa, Y., Grau, D. J., Sarma, K., et al. (2010). Genome-wide identification of polycomb-associated RNAs by RIP-seq. *Molecular Cell*, *40*, 939–953.

Zheng, Y., Sweet, S. M., Popovic, R., Martinez-Garcia, E., Tipton, J. D., Thomas, P. M., et al. (2012). Total kinetic analysis reveals how combinatorial methylation patterns are established on lysines 27 and 36 of histone H3. *Proceedings of the National Academy of Sciences of the United States of America*, *109*, 13549–13554.

Zhou, Z., Gao, J., Popovic, R., Wolniak, K., Parimi, V., Winter, J. N., et al. (2015). Strong expression of EZH2 and accumulation of trimethylated H3K27 in diffuse large B-cell lymphoma independent of cell of origin and EZH2 codon 641 mutation. *Leukemia & Lymphoma*, *56*, 2895–2901.

Zingg, D., Debbache, J., Schaefer, S. M., Tuncer, E., Frommel, S. C., Cheng, P., et al. (2015). The epigenetic modifier EZH2 controls melanoma growth and metastasis through silencing of distinct tumour suppressors. *Nature Communications*, *6*, 6051.

> CHAPTER FOUR

AEG-1/MTDH/LYRIC: A Promiscuous Protein Partner Critical in Cancer, Obesity, and CNS Diseases

L. Emdad[*,†,‡,1], S.K. Das[*,†,‡], B. Hu[*], T. Kegelman[*], D.-c. Kang[§], S.-G. Lee[¶], D. Sarkar[*,†,‡], P.B. Fisher[*,†,‡,1]

[*]Virginia Commonwealth University, School of Medicine, Richmond, VA, United States
[†]VCU Massey Cancer Center, Virginia Commonwealth University, School of Medicine, Richmond, VA, United States
[‡]VCU Institute of Molecular Medicine, Virginia Commonwealth University, School of Medicine, Richmond, VA, United States
[§]Ilsong Institute of Life Science, Hallym University, Anyang, Republic of Korea
[¶]Cancer Preventive Material Development Research Center, Institute of Korean Medicine, College of Korean Medicine, Kyung Hee University, Seoul, Republic of Korea
[1]Corresponding authors: e-mail address: luni.emdad@vcuhealth.org; paul.fisher@vcuhealth.org

Contents

Advances in Cancer Research, Volume 131
ISSN 0065-230X
http://dx.doi.org/10.1016/bs.acr.2016.05.002

Abstract

Since its original discovery in 2002, AEG-1/MTDH/LYRIC has emerged as a primary regulator of several diseases including cancer, inflammatory diseases, and neurodegenerative diseases. AEG-1/MTDH/LYRIC has emerged as a key contributory molecule in almost every aspect of cancer progression, including uncontrolled cell growth, evasion of apoptosis, increased cell migration and invasion, angiogenesis, chemoresistance, and metastasis. Additionally, recent studies highlight a seminal role of AEG-1/MTDH/LYRIC in neurodegenerative diseases and obesity. By interacting with multiple protein partners, AEG-1/MTDH/LYRIC plays multifaceted roles in the pathogenesis of a wide variety of diseases. This review discusses the current state of understanding of AEG-1/MTDH/ LYRIC regulation and function in cancer and other diseases with a focus on its association/interaction with several pivotal protein partners.

1. INTRODUCTION

Astrocyte elevated gene (AEG)-1, also known as metadherin (MTDH) and lysine-rich CEACAM1 coisolated (LYRIC), was originally cloned as an upregulated gene in HIV-1-infected, or TNF-α-treated human astrocytes in 2002 (Hu, Wei, & Kang, 2009; Lee, Kang, DeSalle, Sarkar, & Fisher, 2013; Su et al., 2002; Yoo, Emdad, et al., 2011). Brown and Ruoslahti (2004) cloned mouse AEG-1 using in vivo phage screening, as a protein that facilitated adhesion of mouse 4T1 mammary tumor cells to lung endothelium and named it metadherin (MTDH). Additionally, the mouse/rat ortholog of AEG-1, named lysine-rich CEACAM1 coisolated (LYRIC) (Britt et al., 2004), was cloned as a tight junction protein in polarized rat epithelial cells, and as a novel transmembrane protein (3D3/LYRIC) (Sutherland, Lam, Briers, Lamond, & Bickmore, 2004) located in the endoplasmic reticulum, nuclear envelope, and in the nucleolus. Extensive studies (Huang & Li, 2014; Sarkar & Fisher, 2013; Shi & Wang, 2015; Yoo, Emdad, et al., 2011) have firmly established that AEG-1/MTDH/LYRIC expression is elevated in an wide array of cancers involving almost all parts of the human anatomy, including brain and CNS (glioma, astrocytoma, oligodendroglioma, meningioma, neuroblastoma) (Emdad et al., 2010; He et al., 2014; Hu et al., 2014; Lee et al., 2009, 2011; Liu, Liu, Han, Zhang, & Sun, 2012; Liu et al., 2010; Park et al., 2015; Tong et al., 2016; Xia et al., 2010), GI tract (gastric, esophagus, colorectal, liver, pancreas, gallbladder) (Casimiro et al., 2014; Dong et al., 2015; Gnosa et al., 2012, 2014; Huang et al., 2014; Liu & Yang, 2013; Luo et al., 2015;

Motalleb, Gholipour, & Samaei, 2014; Robertson, Srivastava, Rajasekaran, et al., 2015; Sarkar, 2013; Srivastava et al., 2015; Sun et al., 2011; Yang et al., 2015; Zhu, Liao, He, & Li, 2015), airway system (lung, larynx) (He, He, et al., 2015; Lindskog, Edlund, Mattsson, & Micke, 2015; Liu, Su, et al., 2013; Santarpia et al., 2011; Song et al., 2009), urinary system (prostate, urinary bladder, kidney) (Chen, Ke, Shi, Yang, & Wang, 2010; Erdem, Oktay, Yildirim, Uzunlar, & Kayikci, 2013; Erdem, Yildirim, et al., 2013; Nikpour et al., 2014; Wan, Hu, et al., 2014; Wang, Wei, et al., 2014; Yang et al., 2014), female reproductive system (cervical, ovarian, endometrial) (Haug et al., 2015; Huang, Li, et al., 2013; Li, Chen, et al., 2014; Song, Li, Lu, Zhang, & Geng, 2010), hematopoietic system (leukemia, lymphoma, multiple myeloma) (Gu et al., 2015; Li, Feng, et al., 2015; Li, Feng, et al., 2014; Li, Yao, et al., 2014; Long et al., 2013), head and neck (tongue, salivary gland, oral cavity) (Ke et al., 2013; Li, Wang, Zhao, & Liu, 2015; Liao et al., 2011; Wang, Liu, Chiang, & Wu, 2013), breast (Brown & Ruoslahti, 2004; Hu, chong, et al., 2009; Liu, Zhang, et al., 2011; Tokunaga et al., 2014; Wan & Kang, 2013), skin (melanoma) (Kang et al., 2005), bone (Wang et al., 2011, 2014), etc. One study recently reported the detection of autoantibodies against AEG-1/MTDH/LYRIC in serum samples of several cancer patients including hepatocellular carcinoma (HCC), lung cancer, breast cancer, gastric cancer, and rectal cancer, while AEG-1/MTDH/LYRIC antibody was absent in a large cohorts of normal individual (Chen et al., 2012). Elevated expression of AEG-1/MTDH/LYRIC is regulated by amplification of the gene locus as seen in HCC and breast cancer (Hu, Chong, et al., 2009; Yoo et al., 2009), or through transcriptional regulation by the oncogene c-Myc downstream of the Ha-Ras-PI3K pathway (Lee, Su, Emdad, Sarkar, & Fisher, 2006). Additionally, research over the past several years identified several different miRNAs, which regulate AEG-1/MTDH/LYRIC in different cancers and other diseases. Using gain-of-function and loss-of-function studies and through genetically modified mouse models, it is now confirmed that AEG-1/MTDH/LYRIC controls almost all aspects of cancer aggressiveness by regulating diverse signaling pathways involved in cancer progression and metastasis development (Emdad et al., 2013, 2007; Hu, Wei, et al., 2009; Huang & Li, 2014; Robertson, Srivastava, Rajasekaran, et al., 2015; Robertson et al., 2014; Sarkar, 2013; Sarkar et al., 2009; Shi & Wang, 2015; Yoo, Emdad, et al., 2011). Apart from its seminal role in cancer aggressiveness recent studies also uncovered a potential role of AEG-1/MTDH/LYRIC in obesity (Robertson, Srivastava, Rajasekaran, et al., 2015; Robertson, Srivastava, Siddiq, et al., 2015), which is essentially linked to cancer. Additionally, a detrimental role of AEG-1/MTDH/ LYRIC in neurodegenerative diseases has also been elucidated (Noch & Khalili, 2013). In this chapter, we discuss recent advances providing expanded insights into AEG-1/MTDH/LYRIC regulation and function and also how the protein–protein interactions of AEG-1/MTDH/LYRIC with its interacting protein partners regulate multifaceted processes in cancer and other diseases.

2. REGULATION OF AEG-1/MTDH/LYRIC EXPRESSION

2.1 Induction of AEG-1/MTDH/LYRIC Expression

Evolutionarily, AEG-1/MTDH/LYRIC is highly conserved in mammals and exists only in vertebrates (Lee et al., 2013). AEG-1/MTDH/LYRIC is upregulated in cancer and other diseases by diverse mechanisms, and recent studies are shedding light on the regulatory processes (Fig. 1).

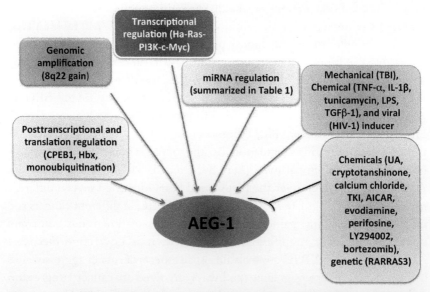

Fig. 1 A model illustrating the diverse regulatory mode of AEG-1/MTDH/LYRIC expression in cancer and other diseases. *CPEB1*, cytoplasmic polyadenylation element-binding protein-1; *Hbx*, hepatitis B viral X protein; *PI3K*, phosphotidylinositol-3-kinase; *TBI*, traumatic brain injury; *TNFα*, tumor necrosis factor α; *(IL)-1β*, interleukin (IL)-1β; *LPS*, lipopolysaccharides; *TGFβ-1*, transforming growth factor β-1; *HIV-1*, human immunodeficiency virus-1; *UA*, ursolic acid; *TKI*, tyrosine kinase inhibitor; *AICAR*, AMP-activated protein kinase (AMPK) activator; *RARRAS3*, retinoic acid receptor responder 3. (See the color plate.)

Included among the diverse regulatory mechanisms that have been identified are genomic amplification, transcriptional regulation, posttranscriptional regulation, and posttranslational regulation. Additionally, several genetic and chemical inducers of AEG-1/MTDH/LYRIC have been identified and validated in recent studies.

2.1.1 Genomic Amplification

Genomic amplification of AEG-1/MTDH/LYRIC has been found in HCC, breast, colorectal, and prostate cancer patients. In HCC, Yoo et al. first documented that AEG-1/MTDH/LYRIC is overexpressed in a large cohort of patients at both mRNA and protein level, and genomic amplification of the AEG-1 locus in chromosome 8q22 was found in a significant percentage of HCC patients (Yoo et al., 2009). Subsequently, another study reported that AEG-1/MTDH/LYRIC was highly amplified in 12.9% of HCCs with a significant *cis*-correlation between somatic copy number, mRNA, and protein expression (Wang, Lim, et al., 2013).

AEG-1/MTDH/LYRIC activation by 8q22 genomic gain has been shown to be an initial event in breast cancer development, which correlated with elevated mRNA and protein expression. Using a computational algorithm, Hu et al. identified the genomic gain of chromosome 8q22, where human AEG-1/MTDH/LYRIC is located (Hu, Chong, et al., 2009). This was further validated in an extensive collection of breast tumor samples and cell lines (Hu, Chong, et al., 2009; Li et al., 2011). In line with these previous reports, another study recently discovered high-level amplifications of AEG-1/MTDH/LYRIC in the primary tumors compared to the metastases (Moelans et al., 2014). Specifically, this study showed a 46% gain in AEG-1/MTDH/LYRIC copy number and 27% amplification in primary (triple negative as well as luminal B) breast tumors. High-level amplification was found in the primary tumor but not in the metastases; however, copy number gain was evident in both primary and metastatic tumors. AEG-1/MTDH/LYRIC was also found to be more frequently amplified in patients with colorectal cancer with relapse to the lung, when compared to patients without lung metastases (Casimiro et al., 2014). In prostate cancer, increased genomic copy number of AEG-1/MTDH/LYRIC was discovered by employing FISH analysis which revealed a significant portion of prostate cancer samples harbored extra genomic copies of the AEG-1/MTDH/LYRIC gene (Wan, Hu, et al., 2014).

2.1.2 Transcriptional Regulation

Lee et al. first reported that AEG-1/MTDH/LYRIC is transcriptionally regulated by c-Myc, which functions downstream of the Ha-Ras-PI3K pathway, suggesting that any disease condition where these components are elevated can result in enhanced expression of AEG-1/MTDH/LYRIC (Lee et al., 2006). Further studies are required to define novel transcriptional regulators of AEG-1/MTDH/LYRIC in cancer and other diseases.

2.1.3 Posttranscriptional and Translational Regulation

In glioma, Kochanek and Wells found that cytoplasmic polyadenylation element-binding protein-1 (CPEB1) can bind to the 3'-UTR of AEG-1/ MTDH/LYRIC mRNA and increases its translation (Kochanek & Wells, 2013). In one recent study the researchers found that hepatitis B viral X protein (HBx) could elevate AEG-1/MTDH/LYRIC protein level without altering its mRNA level (Zhao et al., 2014). Other studies showed that posttranslational regulation of AEG-1/MTDH/LYRIC involves monoubiquitination of protein, which increases its stability and cytoplasmic accumulation in cancer cells (Luxton et al., 2014; Thirkettle, Girling, et al., 2009).

2.1.4 Mechanical and Chemical Inducers

As discussed earlier, AEG-1/MTDH/LYRIC was originally identified as an upregulated gene in human astrocytes infected with HIV-1 (Su et al., 2003, 2002) or treated with HIV-1 gp120 or TNF-α. Using an in vivo mouse model of reactive astrogliosis following mechanical injury Vartak-Sharma & Ghorpade demonstrated increased AEG-1/MTDH/LYRIC expression during astrogliosis (Vartak-Sharma & Ghorpade, 2012). Additionally, in a recent study same research group investigated the role AEG-1/MTDH/ LYRIC in astrocytes responses during HIV-1 infection (Vartak-Sharma, Gelman, Joshi, Borgamann, & Ghorpade, 2014). They found a significant elevated level of AEG-1/MTDH/LYRIC in HIV-1 seropositive (HIV-1+) and HIV-1 encephalitic (HIVE) human brain tissues and also in HIV-1 Tat transgenic mouse brain tissues. They also found a signification induction of AEG-1/MTDH/LYRIC expression when astrocytes were treated with HIV-associated neurocognitive disorders (HAND)-relevant stimuli, including TNF-α, interleukin (IL)-1β, and HIV-1 (Vartak-Sharma et al., 2014). Another study in a Huntington's disease (HD) mouse model, increased AEG-1/ MTDH/LYRIC expression was observed in neurons, following treatment with an ER stress inducer, tunicamycin (Carnemolla et al., 2009). All of these studies associate AEG-1/MTDH/LYRIC as a potent contributor to neuro-inflammatory and neurodegenerative disease pathogenesis. Apart from these inducers, several other inducers of AEG-1/MTDH/LYRIC have also been explored including TGFβ-1 (Wei et al., 2013), compound C—an inhibitor of AMPK (Gollavilli et al., 2015), and lipopolysaccharide (LPS) (Khuda et al., 2009; Zhao et al., 2011).

2.2 Inhibition of AEG-1/MTDH/LYRIC Expression

AEG-1/MTDH/LYRIC has been validated as a *bona fide* oncogene in multiple cancer indications, and no pathological situation to date has been reported where its expression is repressed due to disease. Several recent studies have begun to explore inhibition of AEG-1/MTDH/LYRIC expression as a potential mechanism of anticancer treatment (Fig. 1).

Song et al. first reported that ursolic acid (UA) inhibits AEG-1/MTDH/LYRIC expression in ovarian cancer (Song et al., 2012). Subsequently similar results were reported in lung cancer cells (A549), where the authors found that UA suppressed the expression level of AEG-1/MTDH/LYRIC by repressing nuclear factor-κB signaling (Liu, Guo, et al., 2013). In prostate cancer (Lee et al., 2012), cryptotanshinone was shown to exert its anticancer effects by inhibiting AEG-1/MTDH/LYRIC and HIF-1α. In breast cancer cells, cadmium chloride induced cell death by reducing AEG-1/MTDH/LYRIC expression and NF-κB activity (Luparello, Longo, & Vetrano, 2012). Wang et al. investigated the effects of a multiple tyrosine kinase inhibitor SU6668 in triple negative breast cancer (TNBC) cells and showed that SU6668 inhibits proliferation and redistributes AEG-1/MTDH/LYRIC localization from nuclei to cytoplasm (Wang, Liu, Ma, et al., 2013). Additionally, SU6668 treatment resulted in decreased expression of AEG-1/MTDH/LYRIC, VEGFR2, HIF-1α, and SMA proteins while E-cadherin expression increased. In another study in TNBC, AMP-activated protein kinase (AMPK) activation inhibited AEG-1/MTDH/LYRIC expression, which is partly responsible for its observed anticancer effects (Gollavilli et al., 2015). Interestingly, treatment with AICAR (AMPK activator) or metformin resulted in significant downregulation of its expression via inhibition of c-Myc expression (Gollavilli et al., 2015). The antitumor activity with evodiamine in NSCLC was shown to be partly mediated via inhibition of AEG-1/MTDH/LYRIC expression in A549 cells (Zou et al., 2015). Perifosine, an Akt inhibitor, was shown to have inhibitory effects on the growth of gastric cancer cells (Huang, Yang, et al., 2013). Perifosine decreased AEG-1/MTDH/LYRIC expression along with inhibition of the AKT/GSK3β/c-Myc signaling pathway, which ultimately resulted in inhibition of gastric cancer cell growth (Huang, Yang, et al., 2013). A similar phenomenon was shown in HCC, where the authors investigated the effects of the PI3K inhibitor, LY294002, on regulation of HCC progression and molecular changes (Ma et al., 2014). LY294002 treatment of HCC cells significantly reduced HCC promotion by reducing cell viability, migration, and invasion via downregulation of AEG-1/MTDH/ LYRIC expression, along with suppression of AKT and GSK3β phosphorylation, and expression of their downstream effectors (Ma et al., 2014). A very recent study (Gu et al., 2015) showed that Bortezomib suppressed pre- and posttranscription levels of AEG-1/MTDH/LYRIC expression of multiple myeloma cells in vitro and in vivo.

Aside from these chemical inhibitors of AEG-1/MTDH/LYRIC a genetic repressor has also been reported (Wang, Wang, Hu, et al., 2015). Retinoic acid receptor responder 3 (RARRES3), also known as RIGI, was shown to be significantly downregulated in colorectal cancer tissue and was able to suppress the metastasis of CRC both in vitro and in vivo. Gain-of-function and loss-of-function studies established that RARRES3 is a negative regulator of AEG-1/MTDH/LYRIC (Wang, Wang, Hu, et al., 2015). Although several chemical inhibitors were discovered, additional studies are required to understand the detailed mechanisms of precisely how AEG-1/MTDH/LYRIC is being regulated by these agents.

2.3 miRNA Regulation of AEG-1/MTDH/LYRIC Expression

Studies first reported in 2011 and later have identified miRNAs directly targeting AEG-1/MTDH/LYRIC. Several tumor suppressor miRNAs, which are downregulated in numerous cancers (either overlapping or distinct among various cancers), are considered as upstream regulators of AEG-1/MTDH/LYRIC (summarized in Table 1). In breast cancer, miR-26a was identified as a regulator of AEG-1/MTDH/LYRIC expression, and subsequently the same regulation was found in TNBCs (Liu et al., 2015; Zhang et al., 2011). AEG-1/MTDH/LYRIC was also validated as a target of miRs-30a, -153, -375, and -630 in breast cancer (Li, Zhai, et al., 2015; Ward et al., 2013; Zhang et al., 2014; Zhou et al., 2015). In HCC, several miRNAs were identified as modulators of AEG-1/MTDH/LYRIC 'including miRs-375, -302c, -136, -30a-5p, and -497 (He et al., 2012; Li, Dai, et al., 2015; Yan et al., 2015; Zhao et al., 2014; Zhu et al., 2014).

Table 1 Summary of the miRNAs Regulating AEG-1/MTDH/LYRIC

miRNA	Cancer Types	References
miR-26a	Breast Cancer, TNBC	Zhang et al. (2011) and Liu et al. (2015)
miR-375	Head and neck squamous cell carcinoma	Nohata et al. (2011)
miR-375	Hepatocellular carcinoma	He et al. (2012) and Zhao et al. (2014)
miR-375	Breast cancer	Ward et al. (2013)
miR-375	Esophageal squamous cell carcinoma	Isozaki et al. (2012)
miR-136	Glioma	Yang et al. (2012) and Wu et al. (2014)
miR-30d	Renal cell carcinoma	Wu et al. (2013)
miR-30a	Breast cancer	Zhang et al. (2014)
miR-137	Ovarian cancer	Guo, Xia, Meng, and Lou (2013)
miR-302c	Hepatocellular carcinoma	Zhu et al. (2014)
miR-136	Hepatocellular carcinoma	Zhao et al. (2014)
miR-22	Gastric cancer	Tang et al. (2015)
miR-145	Serous ovarian carcinoma	Dong et al. (2014)
miR-30c	Lung cancer	Suh et al. (2014)
miR-145	Lung cancer	Wang, Shen, et al. (2015), Wang, Wang, Deng, et al. (2015), Wang, Wei, et al. (2015), and Wang, Wang, Hu, et al. (2015)
miR-153	Breast cancer	Li, Feng, et al. (2015), Li, Zhai, Zhao, and Lv (2015), Li, Dai, Ou, Zuo, and Liu (2015), and Li, Wang, et al. (2015)
miR-375	Aldosterone-producing adenoma	He, Cao, et al. (2015) and He, He, et al. (2015)
miR-302c-3p	Glioma	Wang, Shen, et al. (2015), Wang, Wang, Deng, et al. (2015), Wang, Wei, et al. (2015), and Wang, Wang, Hu, et al. (2015)

Continued

Table 1 Summary of the miRNAs Regulating AEG-1/MTDH/LYRIC—cont'd

miRNA	Cancer Types	References
miR-30a-5p	Hepatocellular carcinoma	Li, Feng, et al. (2015), Li, Zhai, Zhao, and Lv (2015), Li, Dai, Ou, Zuo, and Liu (2015), and Li, Wang, et al. (2015)
miR-630	Breast cancer	Zhou et al. (2015)
miR-542-3p	Gastric cancer	Shen et al. (2015)
miR-217	Colorectal cancer	Wang, Shen, et al. (2015), Wang, Wang, Deng, et al. (2015), Wang, Wei, et al. (2015), and Wang, Wang, Hu, et al. (2015)
miR-497	Hepatocellular carcinoma	Yan et al. (2015)

In NSCLC two miRNAs involved in targeting AEG-1/MTDH/LYRIC have been identified so far including miR-30c and -145 (Suh et al., 2014; Wang, Wang, Deng, et al., 2015). AEG-1/MTDH/LYRIC was identified as a target of miRs-136 and -302c-3p in glioma (Wang, Wei, et al., 2015; Wu et al., 2014; Yang et al., 2012). Additionally, miR-375 in HNSCC, EOCC, and aldosterone-producing adenoma (He, Cao, et al., 2015; Isozaki et al., 2012; Nohata et al., 2011; Yan, Lin, & He, 2014), miR-217 in CRC (Wang, Shen, et al., 2015), miR-542-3p and miR-22 in gastric cancer (Shen et al., 2015; Tang et al., 2015), miR-30d in RCC (Wu et al., 2013), and miR-137 and miR-145 in ovarian cancer were shown as regulators of AEG-1/MTDH/LYRIC (Dong et al., 2014; Guo et al., 2013).

3. INTERACTING PARTNERS OF AEG-1/MTDH/LYRIC IN VARIOUS CANCERS

3.1 Interactions Facilitate Cancer Progression by Positively Regulating Tumor-Promoting Genes

AEG-1/MTDH/LYRIC lacks any distinguishable functional domains, which poses an impediment toward understanding the mechanistic basis of its diverse functions. The mainstay of AEG-1/MTDH/LYRIC functions is forming multimeric protein complexes by interacting with several key proteins involved in oncogenesis in multiple subcellular compartments (Fig. 2). A significant advance was made in the past several years in

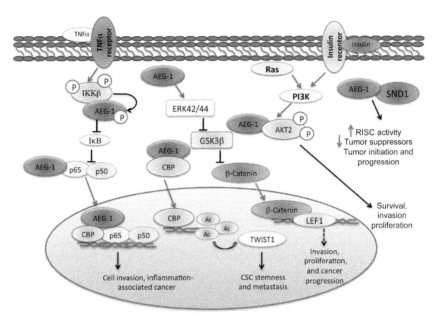

Fig. 2 Schematic diagram of AEG-1/MTDH/LYRIC protein interaction with various tumor-promoting proteins. *Dashed line* indicates pathways yet to be fully characterized. *TNFα*, tumor necrosis factor α; *IKKβ*, I-kappa-β kinaseβ; IκB, inhibitor of κB; *CBP*, cyclic AMP-responsive element-binding protein (CREB)-binding protein; *ERK42/44*, extracellular signal-regulated kinase 42/44; *GSK3β*, glycogen synthase kinase 3β; *Ac*, acetylation; *LEF1*, lymphoid enhancing factor-1; *PI3K*, phosphotidylinositol-3-kinase; *SND1*, staphylococcal nuclease domain-containing 1; RISC, RNA-induced silencing complex. (See the color plate.)

identifying various interacting protein partners of AEG-1/MTDH/LYRIC involved in cancer progression that are discussed in detail in Section 3.1.

3.1.1 NF-κB-p65 and CBP

NF-κB, one of the key signaling pathways involved in AEG-1/MTDH/LYRIC-mediated tumor progression, was first reported by our group (Emdad et al., 2006; Sarkar et al., 2008). Basically we showed that AEG-1/MTDH/LYRIC translocates into the nucleus where it interacted with the p65 subunit of NF-κB and enhanced NF-κB-induced gene expression in HeLa and malignant glioma cells. Subsequently, several studies in diverse cancer indications highlighted the significance of AEG-1/MTDH/LYRIC-mediated NF-κB activation as a key event in oncogenic progression reviewed in Emdad et al. (2013), Huang and Li (2014), Robertson, Srivastava,

Rajasekaran, et al. (2015), Sarkar (2013), Shi and Wang (2015), Wan and Kang (2013), and Yoo, Emdad, et al. (2011). Further evidence emerged from a recent study by (Robertson et al. (2014) in HCC. In this study the authors interrogated the occurrence of DEN-induced HCC in mice lacking AEG-1/MTDH/LYRIC. AEG-1/MTDH/LYRIC genetically ablated mice showed a decreased incidence of HCC and metastatic nodule formation as compared to wild-type mice. Interestingly AEG-1/MTDH/LYRIC-ablated hepatocytes and macrophages displayed a relative defect in NF-κB activation, while no significant difference was observed in other canonical signaling pathways such as AKT, ERK, and β-catenin. These results suggest that AEG-1/MTDH/LYRIC maintains an NF-κB-mediated inflammatory state that facilitates HCC development (Robertson et al., 2014). Another recent study (Krishnan et al., 2015) identified AEG-1/MTDH/LYRIC as a direct substrate of IKKβ. I-kappa-kinase (IKK) complex consists of IKKα, IKKβ, and IKKγ. Activated IKK complex phosphorylates and degrades IκBα proteins (Hayden & Ghosh, 2004), which facilitate nuclear translocation of the NF-κB complex resulting in transcription of specific target genes. To identify new potential substrates of the IKK complex (Krishnan et al., 2015), the authors employed high-resolution mass spectrometry and comprehensive bioinformatics and discovered AEG-1/MTDH/LYRIC as a direct substrate of IKKβ. Following TNF-α activation, IKKβ phosphorylates AEG-1/MTDH/LYRIC on serine 298. They further confirmed that phosphorylation of AEG-1/MTDH/LYRIC is crucial for IκBα degradation as well as NF-κB-dependent gene expression and cell proliferation (Krishnan et al., 2015).

The subcellular localization of AEG-1/MTDH/LYRIC is deemed crucial for its interaction with other partners and functionality, which is regulated by three lysine-rich nuclear localization signal regions (Luxton et al., 2014; Thirkettle, Girling, et al., 2009). One of these regions that is rich in Lysine residues can also be modified by ubiquitin. In a recent paper, Luxton et al. showed that mutation of K486 and K491 residues leads to a significant reduction in AEG-1/MTDH/LYRIC ubiquitination, which then results in altered subcellular distribution and disrupts the interaction between p65 and AEG-1/MTDH/LYRIC (Luxton et al., 2014). A nuclear import chaperone, importin-β, was also confirmed to interact with full length but not with the mutated AEG-1/MTDH/LYRIC. They further identified the potential E3 ligases for the ubiquitination of AEG-1/MTDH/LYRIC and confirmed that the N-terminal fragment of TOPORS interacts with AEG-1/MTDH/LYRIC. In total, this study reveals that specific sites of AEG-1/MTDH/LYRIC ubiquitination are indispensable for regulating AEG-1/MTDH/LYRIC localization and function (Luxton et al., 2014).

Cyclic AMP-responsive element-binding protein (CREB)-binding protein (CBP) and its homolog p300, members of the SRC/p160 family function as coactivator proteins and regulate gene expression by acetylating histones and other transcription factors such as NF-κB (Chen & Greene, 2003). Sarkar et al. first reported that AEG-1/MTDH/LYRIC facilitates NF-κB–CBP complex on the IL-8 promoter in inflammatory responses by interacting with CBP (Sarkar et al., 2008). Inhibition of AEG-1/MTDH/LYRIC by siRNA does not influence NF-κB recruitment but hampers recruitment of CBP to the IL-8 promoter indicating that AEG-1/MTDH/LYRIC functions as a bridging factor among NF-κB, CBP, and the basal transcription machinery (Sarkar et al., 2008). In a recent study, Liang et al. provided further supportive evidence for interaction of AEG-1/MTDH/LYRIC with CBP (Liang et al., 2015). They showed that AEG-1/MTDH/LYRIC controls cancer stem cell (CSC) expansion by regulating a transcription factor important for CSC stemness and metastasis, TWIST1 (Yang et al., 2004). AEG-1/MTDH/LYRIC by interacting with CBP protects it from ubiquitin-mediated degradation and facilitates histone H3 acetylation on the TWIST1 promoter, eventually leading to transcriptional activation of TWIST1 and CSC promotion (Liang et al., 2015).

3.1.2 Staphylococcal Nuclease Domain-Containing Protein 1

Staphylococcal nuclease domain-containing protein 1 (SND1), also known as Tudor staphylococcal nuclease (Tudor-SN) or p100 protein, universally exists in human and many other species (Caudy et al., 2003). SND1 is a component of the RNA-induced silencing complex (RISC) that interacts with Ago-2 to regulate RNA interference (Yoo, Santhekadur, et al., 2011). Additionally, SND1 regulates transcriptional coactivation, mRNA splicing and stability (Yang et al., 2007). Elevated expression of SND1 has been detected in multiple cancer indications, including HCC, breast cancer, prostate cancer, colon cancer, and glioma (Jariwala et al., 2015). Interestingly, SND1 has been identified as an interaction partner of AEG-1/MTDH/LYRIC in some of these malignancies including, HCC, breast cancer, and glioma. Yoo et al. found that both AEG-1/MTDH/LYRIC and SND1 are overexpressed in HCC, and RISC activity was found to be higher in human HCC cells compared to normal hepatocytes (Yoo, Santhekadur, et al., 2011). Employing yeast two-hybrid screening using a human liver

cDNA library and isolation of AEG-1/MTDH/LYRIC-interacting proteins by coimmunoprecipitation followed by mass spectrometry, Yoo
et al. confirmed that AEG-1/MTDH/LYRIC physically interacts with
SND1 via the region 101–205 amino acids (Yoo, Santhekadur, et al.,
2011). Concurrently, Blanco et al. identified SND1 as a candidate AEG-1/
MTDH/LYRIC-interacting protein in breast cancer, which plays an
important role in breast cancer metastasis to the lungs (Blanco et al.,
2011). Additional experiments identified the region of interaction to amino
acids 364–470 of the AEG-1/MTDH/LYRIC coding sequence, which is
very similar to the AEG-1/MTDH/LYRIC lung-homing domain (Blanco
et al., 2011). Two sophisticated studies were then conducted by the same
research group to further understand the mechanistic significance of AEG-1/
MTDH/LYRIC-SND1 interaction in mammary tumorigenesis (Guo
et al., 2014; Wan et al., 2014). In the first study (Wan, Lu, et al., 2014), they
perform a series of experiments using PyMT-AEG-1/MTDH/LYRIC −/−
mammary epithelial cells (MECs). AEG-1/MTDH/LYRIC −/− cells failed
to form mammary sphere formation in vitro and tumor formation in vivo that
was rescued by reintroducing AEG-1/MTDH/LYRIC in these cells. Interestingly, this rescue effect was completely abolished by knocking down
SND1 indicating that AEG-1/MTDH/LYRIC regulates tumor initiation
in cooperation with SND1 (Wan, Lu, et al., 2014). To map the minimal
SND1-binding domain of AEG-1/MTDH/LYRIC, a series of fragments
of AEG-1/MTDH/LYRIC within region 364–582 was generated and tested
for interaction. They found that a 22-amino acid fragment (residues 386–407)
was sufficient for SND1 binding. The authors further showed that AEG-1/
MTDH/LYRIC-SND1 interaction complex is crucial for cell survival
under stress conditions. PyMT-AEG-1/MTDH/LYRIC −/− cells, rec-
onstituted with either WT or mutant mouse AEG-1/MTDH/LYRIC,
treated with camptothecin to induce DNA replication stress conditions.
Interestingly, they found that wt AEG-1/MTDH/LYRIC rescued MECs
from camptothecin-induced apoptosis; however, SND1-binding-deficient
mutations abolished this survival advantage effect of AEG-1/MTDH/
LYRIC (Wan, Lu, et al., 2014). In a subsequent study, Guo et al. identified a short 11-residue peptide in AEG-1/MTDH/LYRIC (residues
393–403) as the primary SND1-binding motif, and SN1/2 domains in
SND1 as AEG-1/MTDH/LYRIC (Guo et al., 2014). They further determined the high-resolution crystal structure of this complex and discovered
a unique interface of AEG-1/MTDH/LYRIC-SND1 interaction that is
essential for the tumor-promoting function of this complex (Guo
et al., 2014).

Another recent study analyzed the expression and potential interaction of AEG-1/MTDH/LYRIC–SND1 in glioma (Tong et al., 2016). They found that both AEG-1/MTDH/LYRIC and SND1 were highly expressed in glioma, and coexpression of AEG-1/MTDH/LYRIC and SND1 was associated with advanced glioma grades. Additionally, they detected the interaction between AEG-1/MTDH/LYRIC and SND1 in cultured glioma cell lines. By additional experiments the authors showed that AEG-1/MTDH/LYRIC might promote glioma by inducing SND1 expression through the activation of NF-κB pathway (Tong et al., 2016). In CRC, a significant correlation was observed between SND1 and AEG-1/MTDH/LYRIC expression that positively correlated with tumor grade and cancer progression (Wang et al., 2012).

The functional dependency of AEG-1/MTDH/LYRIC on its conserved interaction with SND1, together with the observation that systemic deletion of AEG-1/MTDH/LYRIC is well tolerated in mice, suggest that targeting the AEG-1/MTDH/LYRIC-SND1 complex may offer an opportunity to control tumor initiation, recurrence, and metastasis by preventing the expansion of tumor-initiation cells, with minimal impact on normal tissues.

3.1.3 AKT2

AKT (protein kinase B) functions as an essential regulator of cell proliferation, survival, migration, and invasion as a nexus-signaling molecule in the receptor tyrosine kinase/phosphatidylinositol 3-kinase pathway (Burgering & Coffer, 1995). *AKT1*, *AKT2*, and *AKT3* are three homologous isoforms belong to the *AKT* gene. Lee et al. first demonstrated that AEG-1/MTDH/LYRIC functions as a downstream target of *Ha-Ras*, and induction of AEG-1/MTDH/LYRIC was attenuated by treatment with a PI3K inhibitor—LY294002 or phosphatase and tensin homolog overexpression (Lee et al., 2006). In another study, AEG-1/MTDH/LYRIC overexpression inhibited serum starvation-induced apoptosis by activating the *Ras* and PI3K-AKT signaling pathways (Lee, Su, Emdad, Sarkar, et al., 2008). Subsequently, AEG-1/MTDH/LYRIC regulation of AKT signaling pathways was shown to be critical in cell proliferation, invasion, apoptosis resistance, chemoresistance, and angiogenesis in multiple cancer contexts by several groups (Emdad et al., 2013; Sarkar, 2013; Shi & Wang, 2015; Wan & Kang, 2013). However, the mechanism by which AEG-1/MTDH/LYRIC regulated AKT remained unclear.

In one recent study, Hu et al. demonstrated a novel specific interaction between AEG-1/MTDH/LYRIC and AKT2 in glioma (Hu et al., 2014).

They found that AEG-1/MTDH/LYRIC specifically interacts with AKT2 and not with AKT1 or AKT3 isoforms in GBM. Immunohistochemistry analysis and TCGA data analysis revealed a high correlation between expression of AEG-1/MTDH/LYRIC and AKT2 in clinical glioma samples and confirmed the clinical significance of these two key molecules with glioma patient survival. They confirmed that AKT2-PH domain is responsible for interacting with AEG-1/MTDH/LYRIC in glioma and also mapped the interacting regions in AEG-1/MTDH/LYRIC (Hu et al., 2014). AEG-1/MTDH/LYRIC-AKT2 interaction prolonged stabilization of AKT2 phosphorylation at S474 and disruption of this interaction reduced phosphorylation of the proapoptotic protein, Bcl-2-associated death promoter (BAD) and AEG-1/MTDH/LYRIC-mediated invasion gain. Additionally, they showed that conditional expression of AKT2-PH domain combined with AEG-1/MTDH/LYRIC silencing significantly enhanced survival in an orthotopic mouse model of human GBM. These findings highlight the importance of AEG-1/MTDH/LYRIC-AKT2 interaction in glioma proliferation, survival, and invasion and confirm that AEG-1/MTDH/LYRIC-AKT2 is a critical protein–protein signaling complex in glioma (Hu et al., 2014). Further exploring this interaction in other cancer contexts in which both of these molecules are highly upregulated would be very informative and valuable.

3.1.4 Other Interacting Partners: β-Catenin, Ubn-1

3.1.4.1 β-Catenin

In a recent study, a positive correlation between AEG-1/MTDH/LYRIC and β-catenin nuclear expression in CRC was reported (Zhang et al., 2013). Ectopic expression of AEG-1/MTDH/LYRIC robustly increased nuclear β-catenin accumulation in CRC cell lines. Additionally, AEG-1/MTDH/LYRIC interacted with β-catenin in SW480 CRC cells. We recently found that AEG-1/MTDH/LYRIC, β-catenin, and LEF-1 form a protein complex in glioma stem cells (GSC) (B. Hu, L. Emdad, S.K. Das, D. Sarkar, & P.B. Fisher, unpublished observations). LEF-1 has been shown to interact with β-catenin and functions as transcriptional coactivators for Wnt target genes (Huber et al., 1996). Further investigation of the interaction between these three proteins in GSC and other cancer types would be of value.

3.1.4.2 Ubn-1

In a recent study, Lupo et al. identified AEG-1/MTDH/LYRIC as an interacting partner of Ubinuclein (Ubn-1) in epithelial cells (Lupo et al., 2012).

Ubn-1 is a nuclear protein interacting with the EBV transcription factor EB1 and other cellular transcription factor of the leucine-zipper family including C/EBP or Jun. Employing mass spectrometry the authors identified AEG-1/MTDH/LYRIC as a potential binding partner of Ubn-1 and validated it via coimmunoprecipitation and confocal microscopy analyses (Lupo et al., 2012). AEG-1/MTDH/LYRIC and Ubn-1 are colocated at the tight junction in HT29 CRC cells. Further studies are necessary to identify the domains of this interaction and potential role(s) of this interaction in tumorigenesis and/or other disease processes.

3.2 Interactions Facilitate Cancer Progression by Negatively Regulating Tumor Suppressor Genes

Apart from positive regulation of tumor-promoting genes, outlined earlier, AEG-1/MTDH/LYRIC also interacts with several tumor suppressor genes and negatively regulates their functions (Fig. 3). These studies are elaborated below.

3.2.1 Promyelocytic Leukemia Zinc Finger Protein

Using the yeast two-hybrid approach, Thirkettle et al. identified promyelocytic leukemia zinc finger protein (PLZF) as an interacting protein

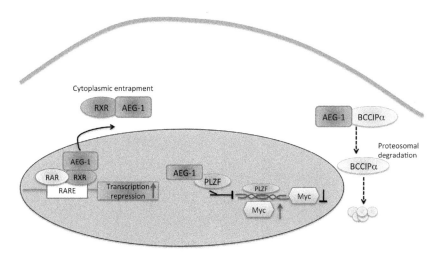

Fig. 3 Schematic diagram of AEG-1/MTDH/LYRIC protein interaction with various tumor suppressor proteins. *Dashed line* indicates pathways yet to be fully characterized. *RxR*, retinoid X receptor; *RAR*, retinoic acid receptor; *RARE*, retinoic acid response elements; *PLZF*, promyelocytic leukemia zinc finger protein; *BCCIPα*, BRCA2- and CDKN1A (p21$^{Cip1/Waf-1/mda-6}$)-associated protein. (See the color plate.)

partner of AEG-1/MTDH/LYRIC (Thirkettle, Mills, Whitaker, & Neal, 2009). Both AEG-1/MTDH/LYRIC and PLZF colocalize to nuclear bodies containing histone deacetylases, which facilitates PLZF-mediated transcriptional repression. Two regions in amino- and carboxyl terminals of AEG-1/MTDH/LYRIC were important for this interaction, namely, 1–285 amino acids in NH_2-terminal and 487–582 amino acids in COOH-terminal (Thirkettle, Mills, et al., 2009). The authors also mapped the region of interaction in PLZF and identified that 322–404 amino acids in PLZF were sufficient to interact with AEG-1/MTDH/LYRIC. This region in PLZF contains two lysine residues verified to be crucial for PLZF activation by SUMOylation. The authors mutated the key lysine (K242R) residue responsible for PLZF SUMOylation and showed that AEG-1/MTDH/LYRIC failed to interact with the mutated PLZF further indicating that AEG-1/MTDH/LYRIC only interacts with the active form of PLZF (Thirkettle, Mills, et al., 2009). PLZF is a transcriptional repressor and associated with growth suppression and apoptosis by transcriptionally regulating many genes including c-Myc. Interaction of AEG-1/MTDH/LYRIC with PLZF precludes its recruitment to the c-Myc promoter, thereby resulting in increased transcription of c-Myc (Thirkettle, Mills, et al., 2009). This study provides a new mechanism explaining how AEG-1/MTDH/LYRIC functions as an oncogene by blocking PLZF's repressive functions on gene transcription.

3.2.2 BRCA2- and CDKN1A (p21$^{Cip1/Waf-1/mda-6}$)-Associated Protein (BCCIPα)

In prostate cancer, Ash et al. identified BCCIPα as an AEG-1/MTDH/LYRIC-interacting protein using a yeast two-hybrid screen (Ash, Yang, & Britt, 2008). Reduced expression of BCCIPα has been documented in breast cancer and glioma and ectopic expression of BCCIPα caused growth delay in these cancers, suggesting that BCCIPα plays a suppressive role in tumorigenesis. BCCIPα also functions in cell cycle regulation by binding to p21 (MDA-6) and enhances p21-mediated Cdk2 kinase inhibition (Ash et al., 2008). When AEG-1/MTDH/LYRIC was coexpressed with BCCIPα in prostate cancer cells, it caused a decrease in BCCIPα protein levels, suggesting that AEG-1/MTDH/LYRIC may serve as a possible negative regulator of BCCIPα. The authors further mapped the interaction region of AEG-1/MTDH/LYRIC–BCCIPα and found that amino acids 72–192 of AEG-1/MTDH/LYRIC are important for this interaction (Ash et al., 2008). However, the functional role of BCCIPα degradation in mediating AEG-1/MTDH/LYRIC function remains to be elucidated.

3.2.3 Retinoid X Receptor

Retinoid X Receptor (RXR) is an important member of the nuclear receptor superfamily and it functions via homodimerization with itself or several other nuclear receptors (Mangelsdorf, Ong, Dyck, & Evans, 1990). Altered expression and function of RXR has been reported as a contributing factor in the development of many cancers and other diseases (Szanto et al., 2004). One recent study by Srivastava et al. identified RXR as an interacting partner of AEG-1/MTDH/LYRIC in HCC (Srivastava et al., 2014). When AEG-1/MTDH/LYRIC interacts with RXR it significantly impairs its transcriptional activation ability. Interestingly, in normal hepatocytes AEG-1/MTDH/LYRIC-RXR colocated in the nucleus; however, in tumor cells this interaction complex was restricted to the cytoplasm (Srivastava et al., 2014). In the absence of ligand, the RXR/RAR complex binds to target gene promoters and recruits corepressor complex; however, in the presence of ligand it recruits coactivators and regulates target gene transcription involved in normal cell proliferation and apoptosis. While in complex with RXR in the normal cell nuclei, AEG-1/MTDH/LYRIC interferes with coactivator recruitment. However, in cancer cells where AEG-1/MTDH/LYRIC expression is elevated and accumulates in the cytoplasm, it entraps RXR in the cytoplasm and hampers transcriptional activation of target genes (Srivastava et al., 2014). Additionally, the negative regulation of AEG-1/MTDH/LYRIC also occurred via phosphorylation of RXR. The authors also mapped the regions of interaction in both molecules and found that 1–70 amino acids in the amino terminal region of AEG-1/MTDH/LYRIC, particularly the LXXLL motif, are crucial for the interaction with RXR, and the ligand-binding domain of RXR is important in mediating its interaction with AEG-1/MTDH/LYRIC (Srivastava et al., 2014). Fundamentally, AEG-1/MTDH/LYRIC upregulation results in RXRs inactivation, thereby negatively affecting downstream signaling and facilitating uncontrolled cancer cell proliferation leading to HCC and other cancers.

In summary, although initially based on its putative gene/amino acid sequence, the molecular basis of AEG-1/MTDH/LYRIC action remained somewhat ambiguous the observation that AEG-1/MTDH/LYRIC's *modus operandi* involves protein–protein interactions has expanded our appreciation of the mechanism(s) of action of this intriguing molecule. These interactions are indispensible for AEG-1/MTDH/LYRIC regulation of cancer cell phenotypes, and disrupting the interaction of AEG-1/MTDH/LYRIC with its specific diverse partner proteins may prove useful for cancer therapeutics. However, further studies are required to illuminate how AEG-1/MTDH/LYRIC selects its interacting partners and interrupts protein degradation in order to enable feasibility of such approaches.

4. AEG-1/MTDH/LYRIC: ROLE IN OBESITY

Obesity is essentially linked to fatty liver disease, heart disease, cancer, and other diseases (Font-Burgada, Sun, & Karin, 2016). A recent study underscores a novel role of AEG-1/MTDH/LYRIC in lipid metabolism and obesity (Robertson, Srivastava, Siddiq, et al., 2015). In this study Robertson et al. generated and characterized an AEG-1 knockout (AEG-1KO) mouse, which was viable and fertile. Interestingly, the AEG-1KO mouse was skinny as compared to a wild-type mouse even with a similar level of food consumption. MRI analysis revealed a significant decrease in subcutaneous, visceral, and intramuscular fat in the AEG-1KO mice compared with WT mice (Robertson, Srivastava, Siddiq, et al., 2015). As the mice aged the WT mice developed fatty changes in their livers, while these changes were not evident in the AEG-1/MTDH/LYRIC KO group.

AEG-1KO mice fed a high fat and cholesterol diet did not gain any significant weight, whereas rapid weight gain was observed in WT mice. Failure of weight gain in AEG-1KO mice was due to decreased fat absorption from the intestines, with no significant changes in fat synthesis or fat consumption. Additional mechanistic studies revealed that lack of AEG-1/MTDH/LYRIC in mice augmented LXR and PPARα activity, which are the major inhibitors of intestinal fat absorption (Robertson, Srivastava, Siddiq, et al., 2015). AEG-1KO mice live significantly longer than WT mice perhaps due to the natural inability of AEG-1KO mice to accumulate fat. These studies discover a novel role of AEG-1/MTDH/LYRIC in maintaining homeostasis in lipid metabolism further emphasizing its significance as a therapeutic target in obesity-associated cancers and other diseases.

5. AEG-1/MTDH/LYRIC AND CNS DISEASE

Besides AEG-1/MTDH/LYRIC's role as a prominent oncogene and essential component in regulating diverse cellular signaling pathways, several recent studies highlight a central role of AEG-1/MTDH/LYRIC in central nervous disease pathogenesis (reviewed in Kim et al., 2011;

Noch & Khalili, 2013). Contributions of AEG-1/MTDH/LYRIC have been reported in HIV-1-associated neuroinflammation, neurodegenerative diseases such as HD and amyotrophic lateral sclerosis (ALS), migraine, reactive astrogliosis, and glioma-associated neurodegeneration, which are discussed in detail below.

5.1 HIV-1-Associated Neuroinflammation

AEG-1/MTDH/LYRIC was initially discovered and isolated from HIV-1-infected human fetal astrocytes and later confirmed as an established oncogene in many cancer indications; however, its role in HIV-1-associated neurological pathology has just begun to be explored in detail. In a recent study, Vartak-Sharma et al. investigated the changes in AEG-1/MTDH/LYRIC expression in HIV-1-infected brain tissues and revealed a potential function of AEG-1/MTDH/LYRIC in HAND (Vartak-Sharma et al., 2014). They compared the expression of AEG-1/MTDH/LYRIC in cell lysates from frontal cortex of 12 HIV-1+, 11 HIVE, and 12 age-, race-, and gender-matched control subjects. Additionally, they included HIV-1 Tat transgenic (GT-tg) mouse brain tissues in these sample groups. They found that AEG-1/MTDH/LYRIC expression was significantly elevated in HIV-1+, and HIVE samples as compared to control group and GT-tg mouse brain tissues also exhibited higher AEG-1/MTDH/LYRIC expression as compared to WT mouse brain (Vartak-Sharma et al., 2014). Cultured astrocytes expressing HIV-1 Tat similarly showed high AEG-1/MTDH/LYRIC and cytokine expression. Furthermore, astrocytes treated with HAND-relevant stimuli, including TNF-α, IL-1β, or HIV-1, significantly induced AEG-1/MTDH/LYRIC expression and nuclear translocation via activation of the NF-κB pathway (Vartak-Sharma et al., 2014). They further demonstrated that AEG-1/MTDH/LYRIC interacted with NF-κB-p65, in both naïve and activated astrocytes. In unstimulated astrocytes, NF-κB-p65 exists in a complex with AEG-1/MTDH/LYRIC in the cell cytoplasm; in response to TNF-α, this complex translocates to the nucleus. Furthermore, treatment with IL-1β resulted in decreased expression of excitatory amino acid transporter 2 (EAAT2), increased expression of EAAT2 repressor ying yang 1 (YY1), and reduced glutamate clearance in AEG-1/MTDH/LYRIC-overexpressed astrocytes. This study identified a novel function of AEG-1/MTDH/LYRIC in the pathogenesis of astrocyte-driven neuroinflammatory processes in patients with HAND (Vartak-Sharma et al., 2014).

5.2 Neurodegenerative Diseases Such as HD and ALS

HD is an inherited autosomal-dominant neurodegenerative disorder caused by a CAG repeat expansion of the HD gene, which encodes for Huntington protein. In a recent study Carnemolla et al. demonstrated that regulator of ribosome synthesis (Rrs1), a differentially regulated gene in HD, is localized both in the nucleolus as well as in the ER of neurons from a knock-in mouse model of HD (Carnemolla et al., 2009). The authors found that AEG-1/MTDH/LYRIC interacted with Rrs1 and shared its dual-subcellular localization in the ER and nucleolus. Immunohistochemical analysis of HD brains revealed a ~1.7-fold-upregulated expression of AEG-1/MTDH/LYRIC over control brains, indicating that this overexpression may be associated with the pathogenesis of HD. These data imply that both Rrs1 and AEG-1/MTDH/LYRIC might function as an ER stress sensor in HD and participate in transducing these signals to the nucleolus (Carnemolla et al., 2009).

ALS is a rapid, progressive neurodegenerative disease with indistinct etiology. Degeneration of the motor neurons is a major characteristic of the pathological features in ALS. In a recent study AEG-1/MTDH/LYRIC expression was markedly downregulated in motor neurons from an in vivo mouse model as well as cell culture models of ALS at both mRNA and protein levels (Yin et al., 2015). Upon silencing of AEG-1/MTDH/LYRIC in NSC34 cells a significant reduction in cell viability in association with PI3K/AKT signaling pathways was apparent as evidenced by reduced p-Akt, p-GSK-3β, and p-PDK1 levels. Additional experiments revealed that p-CREB was reduced in mSOD1 cells, and both a PI3K activator and lithium could upregulate the expression of p-CREB and AEG-1/MTDH/LYRIC. In essence this study implies that reduced AEG-1/MTDH/LYRIC expression, in association with PI3K/Akt/CREB pathway inhibition, establishes a negative feedback in ALS motor neurons, resulting in their death (Yin et al., 2015).

5.3 Migraine

Migraine is one of the common neurological disorders usually associated with repeated attacks of headache and other symptoms like photophobia, nausea, and vomiting. Two main subgroups of migraine are described: migraine with aura (MA) and migraine without aura (MO). A few recently published genome-wide association studies (GWAS) using data from migraine patients found evidence for a role of the AEG-1/MTDH/LYRIC gene in common migraine (Anttila et al., 2010; Anttila, Wessman, Kallela, & Palotie, 2011; Freilinger et al., 2012; Ligthart et al., 2011; Ran et al., 2014). Anttila et al. first identified an association of a single nucleotide polymorphism (SNP) rs1835740 on 8q22.1 with migraine in a two-stage GWAS provided by seven North European migraine populations (Anttila et al., 2010). The SNP rs1835740 is located in a 27-kb haplotype block between two interesting candidate genes: AEG-1/MTDH/LYRIC and the plasma glutamate carboxypeptidase. Furthermore, an expression quantitative trait locus analysis revealed that the rs1835740 risk allele was associated with higher AEG-1/MTDH/LYRIC expression (Anttila et al., 2010). AEG-1/MTDH/LYRIC was also recently found to be associated with migraine in a genome-wide meta-analysis including six population-based European cohorts (Ligthart et al., 2011). Another GWAS was performed on German and Dutch migraine patients without aura, and this study found associations with four new loci (Freilinger et al., 2012). Finally, a more recent study analyzed eight SNPs in a Swedish cohort previously identified with genetic risk factors for migraine in a European GWAS: rs2651899 (1p36.32), rs3790455 (1q22), rs10166942 (2q37.1), rs7640543 (3p24), rs9349379 (6p24), rs1835740 (8q22), rs6478241 (9p33), and rs11172113 (12q13.3) (Ran et al., 2014). Similar to the previous European cohorts a trend was observed for association of rs1835740 with migraine in a population-based cohort including migraine patients both with and without aura. However, further association of AEG-1/MTDH/LYRIC was not investigated in this Swedish cohort of migraine patients that might be worth following in the future.

5.4 Reactive Astrogliosis

CNS insults such as trauma, infection, neurodegeneration, and post-neurosurgical healing are often linked to reactive astrogliosis. In a recent study, the authors (Vartak-Sharma and Ghorpade) utilized an in vivo brain injury mouse model of reactive astrogliosis and identified AEG-1/MTDH/LYRIC as a novel regulator in mediating reactive astrogliosis (Vartak-Sharma & Ghorpade, 2012). In particular, they showed induction of AEG-1/MTDH/LYRIC in astrocytes at the injury sites and AEG-1/MTDH/LYRIC localized to the astrocyte nucleolus. Further experiments indicated that AEG-1/MTDH/LYRIC facilitates wound healing by regulating proliferation and migration of astrocytes. These results indicate a role of AEG-1/MTDH/LYRIC in mediating reactive astrogliosis as well as in regulating astrocyte responses to brain injury (Vartak-Sharma & Ghorpade, 2012). The association of AEG-1/MTDH/LYRIC during reactive astrogliosis has uncovered multiple possibilities to investigate neuropathology; however, further studies are required to achieve a better understanding of its role in this CNS pathology.

5.5 Glioma-Associated Neurodegeneration

Glutamate is the major excitatory amino acid transmitter in the mammalian CNS and excess glutamate exposure leads to neuronal death through excitotoxicity (Kim et al., 2011; Lee et al., 2013). Among the five excitatory amino acid transporters (EAAT 1–5), EAAT2 is the most abundant glutamate transporter in brain, which plays an important role in balancing the glutamate concentration at physiologically low level (Lee, Su, Emdad, Gupta, et al., 2008; Rothstein et al., 2005). Impaired glutamate uptake by glial cells causes excitotoxicity, which has been associated with various neurodegenerative disease conditions such as epilepsy, stroke, ALS, traumatic brain injury, HIV-associated dementia, and also in some psychiatric disorders like depression and schizophrenia (Noch & Khalili, 2013). Kang et al. originally documented an inverse correlation between EAAT2 and AEG-1/MTDH/LYRIC expression (Kang et al., 2005). A recent study by Lee et al. further expanded the initial observation and found a strong negative correlation between expression of AEG-1/MTDH/LYRIC and EAAT2 in normal brain tissues and glioma patient samples (Lee et al., 2011). At the molecular level, AEG-1/MTDH/LYRIC directly interacts with YY-1 and CBP and functions as a bridge molecule between YY1 and CBP and the basal transcription machinery. This ultimately caused YY1 to function as a negative regulator of EAAT2 expression by inhibiting CBP. AEG-1/MTDH/LYRIC-mediated EAAT2 repression resulted in reduction of glutamate uptake by glial cells and induction of neuronal cell death, thus contributing to glioma-induced neurodegeneration (Lee et al., 2011).

6. AEG-1/MTDH/LYRIC: ROLE IN INFECTION AND INFLAMMATION

A novel role of AEG-1/MTDH/LYRIC has also been described in viral infectivity. Specifically, the authors have shown that HIV-1 Gag and AEG-1/MTDH/LYRIC make an interaction complex, and this interaction was also observed in equine infectious anemia virus and murine leukemia virus, suggesting that it represents a conserved feature among retroviruses (Engeland et al., 2011). Expression of an AEG-1/MTDH/LYRIC mutant lacking the Gag-binding region resulted in lower Gag expression and decreased viral infectivity. Further insights into the role of AEG-1/ MTDH/LYRIC in viral infectivity came from studying dengue virus, which revealed AEG-1/MTDH/LYRIC facilitates viral spread via enhancing vascular permeability (Liu, Chiu, Chen, & Wu, 2011). AEG-1/ MTDH/LYRIC has also recently been shown to be linked to the regulation of inflammation and immune responses (Gong et al., 2012; Huang, Li, et al., 2013; Li, Wang, et al., 2014; Robertson et al., 2014; Vartak-Sharma et al., 2014). Recent clinical and epidemiologic studies strongly linked chronic infection and inflammation to cancer initiation and progression (Shalapour & Karin, 2015). Correlations have been found between HCC and chronic viral hepatitis, and HPV infection and cervical cancer, *H. pylori* infection in gastric cancer and inflammatory bowel disease with colon cancer and in all these cancer indications AEG-1/MTDH/LYRIC has emerged as an important contributor for disease pathogenesis (Gong et al., 2012; Li, Wang, et al., 2014; Luo et al., 2015; Yoo et al., 2009). It is worth further investigating the significance of deregulated AEG-1/ MTDH/LYRIC expression in infection- and inflammation-associated conditions.

7. CONCLUSIONS AND FUTURE PERSPECTIVES

In the past decade, remarkable advances have been made in deciphering the multidimensional roles of AEG-1/MTDH/LYRIC in the regulation of cancers and other disease processes (Huang & Li, 2014; Meng, Thiel, & Leslie, 2013; Noch & Khalili, 2013; Sarkar, 2013; Wan & Kang, 2013). In the oncology arena, AEG-1/MTDH/LYRIC is now considered to be a potential biomarker for more aggressive cancers (Sarkar & Fisher, 2013; Shi & Wang, 2015). However, further extensive studies in large cohorts of patients and correlative studies with clinical parameters are necessary to establish this gene as a screening tool for cancer diagnosis. Stringent quality control is necessary to detect AEG-1/MTDH/LYRIC mRNA/ protein in blood, urine, and other body fluid, and in biopsy samples, and comparative studies are required to verify its specificity and sensitivity vs other currently employed serum biomarkers. Another exciting use of the AEG-1/MTDH/LYRIC gene (its promoter) for cancer detection was recently described using imaging reporter gene construct under the control of its promoter and a nanoparticle-based delivery method (Bhatnagar et al., 2014). In this study, Bhatnagar et al. used a clinically relevant bone metastatic model of prostate cancer and was successfully able to detect malignant lesions using nanoparticle-delivered AEG-Prom construct through bioluminescence imaging and single-photon emission computed tomography (Bhatnagar et al., 2014). This observation suggests that AEG-1/MTDH/LYRIC promoter is a useful tool to detect cancer lesions in a minimally invasive manner and uncovers additional avenues to investigate which will impact its utility in other cancer contexts. As a functional perspective, AEG-1/MTDH/LYRIC is established as an important mediator of cancer development and progression via regulation of several key processes of tumorigenesis including uncontrolled growth promotion, evasion of apoptosis, invasion, and migration, angiogenesis, chemoresistance, and metastasis. To gain an expanded understanding on the precise mechanism of action of this multifunctional gene in vivo, knockout and transgenic animal models represent highly beneficial research tools. Recent developments with hepatocyte-specific transgenic mice expressing AEG-1/MTDH/LYRIC (albumin (Alb)/AEG-1), c-Myc (Alb/c-Myc), or both (Alb/AEG-1/c-Myc) and AEG-1-knockout mice revealed novel aspects of AEG-1/MTDH/LYRIC functions that might not have been possible by simply using nude mice xenograft studies. In these contexts, developing additional conditional transgenic animal models using tissue-specific targeted expression of AEG-1/MTDH/LYRIC and crossing these with other tumor models will significantly expand our understanding of AEG-1/MTDH/LYRIC functions in additional cancer indications.

The ability of AEG-1/MTDH/LYRIC to interact with a significant number of proteins (discussed in detail in this review), thereby regulating their stability and functions is of immense interest for future research. Furthermore, the biochemical modifications occurring to AEG-1/MTDH/LYRIC itself is worthy of further investigation. Information garnered from both of these endeavors may aid in developing optimal inhibitors or therapeutic drugs against cancer or other diseases where aberrant expression of AEG-1/MTDH/LYRIC had been observed. Small molecules that disrupt AEG-1/MTDH/LYRIC interactions with their binding partners can be determined using high-throughput screening combined with NMR. Additionally, unraveling the crystal structure of protein–protein interaction domains may facilitate the in silico design of putative small molecule inhibitors of AEG-1/MTDH/LYRIC. In this context, a study by Guo et al.

which determined the crystal structure of the AEG-1/MTDH/LYRIC-SND1 complex is a good beginning that requires further exploration (Guo et al., 2014).

In summary, in this review we discuss recent insights on AEG-1/MTDH/LYRIC regulation and function in diverse disease contexts. We have made significant inroads in understanding this exciting molecule. However, more extensive research is warranted and should lead to a greater comprehension of physiological and pathological functions of this protein, which may aid in developing targeted therapeutics in various pathogenic diseases, including cancer, CNS disease, obesity-associated diseases and other clinically relevant disease states.

ACKNOWLEDGMENTS

The present studies were supported in part by NIH NCI R01 CA134721 (Fisher), P50 CA058236 (Pomper and Fisher), The Prostate Cancer Foundation A. David Mazzone-PCF Challenge Award (Pomper, Fisher and Sguoros), and the National Foundation for Cancer Research (Fisher). Dr. Fisher is cofounder of, serves as a consultant, and has ownership interest in Cancer Targeting Systems (CTS), Inc. Virginia Commonwealth University, Johns Hopkins University, and Columbia University have ownership interest in CTS, Inc.

REFERENCES

Anttila, V., Stefansson, H., Kallela, M., Todt, U., Terwindt, G. M., Calafato, M. S., et al. (2010). Genome-wide association study of migraine implicates a common susceptibility variant on 8q22.1. *Nature Genetics, 42,* 869–873.

Anttila, V., Wessman, M., Kallela, M., & Palotie, A. (2011). Towards an understanding of genetic predisposition to migraine. *Genome Medicine, 3,* 17.

Ash, S. C., Yang, D. Q., & Britt, D. E. (2008). LYRIC/AEG-1 overexpression modulates BCCIPalpha protein levels in prostate tumor cells. *Biochemical and Biophysical Research Communications, 371,* 333–338.

Bhatnagar, A., Wang, Y., Mease, R. C., Gabrielson, M., Sysa, P., Minn, I., et al. (2014). AEG-1 promoter-mediated imaging of prostate cancer. *Cancer Research, 74,* 5772–5781.

Blanco, M. A., Aleckovic, M., Hua, Y., Li, T., Wei, Y., Xu, Z., et al. (2011). Identification of staphylococcal nuclease domain-containing 1 (SND1) as a metadherin-interacting protein with metastasis-promoting functions. *The Journal of Biological Chemistry, 286,* 19982–19992.

Britt, D. E., Yang, D. F., Yang, D. Q., Flanagan, D., Callanan, H., Lim, Y. P., et al. (2004). Identification of a novel protein, LYRIC, localized to tight junctions of polarized epithelial cells. *Experimental Cell Research, 300,* 134–148.

Brown, D. M., & Ruoslahti, E. (2004). Metadherin, a cell surface protein in breast tumors that mediates lung metastasis. *Cancer Cell, 5,* 365–374.

Burgering, B. M., & Coffer, P. J. (1995). Protein kinase B (c-Akt) in phosphatidylinositol-3-OH kinase signal transduction. *Nature, 376,* 599–602.

Carnemolla, A., Fossale, E., Agostoni, E., Michelazzi, S., Calligaris, R., De Maso, L., et al. (2009). Rrs1 is involved in endoplasmic reticulum stress response in Huntington disease. *The Journal of Biological Chemistry, 284,* 18167–18173.

Casimiro, S., Fernandes, A., Oliveira, A. G., Franco, M., Pires, R., Peres, M., et al. (2014). Metadherin expression and lung relapse in patients with colorectal carcinoma. *Clinical & Experimental Metastasis*, *31*, 689–696.

Caudy, A. A., Ketting, R. F., Hammond, S. M., Denli, A. M., Bathoorn, A. M., Tops, B. B., et al. (2003). A micrococcal nuclease homologue in RNAi effector complexes. *Nature*, *425*, 411–414.

Chen, X., Dong, K., Long, M., Lin, F., Wang, X., Wei, J., et al. (2012). Serum anti-AEG-1 auto-antibody is a potential novel biomarker for malignant tumors. *Oncology Letters*, *4*, 319–323.

Chen, L. F., & Greene, W. C. (2003). Regulation of distinct biological activities of the NF-kappaB transcription factor complex by acetylation. *Journal of Molecular Medicine (Berlin, Germany)*, *81*, 549–557.

Chen, W., Ke, Z., Shi, H., Yang, S., & Wang, L. (2010). Overexpression of AEG-1 in renal cell carcinoma and its correlation with tumor nuclear grade and progression. *Neoplasma*, *57*, 522–529.

Dong, R., Liu, X., Zhang, Q., Jiang, Z., Li, Y., Wei, Y., et al. (2014). miR-145 inhibits tumor growth and metastasis by targeting metadherin in high-grade serous ovarian carcinoma. *Oncotarget*, *5*, 10816–10829.

Dong, L., Qin, S., Li, Y., Zhao, L., Dong, S., Wang, Y., et al. (2015). High expression of astrocyte elevated gene-1 is associated with clinical staging, metastasis, and unfavorable prognosis in gastric carcinoma. *Tumour Biology*, *36*, 2169–2178.

Emdad, L., Das, S. K., Dasgupta, S., Hu, B., Sarkar, D., & Fisher, P. B. (2013). AEG-1/MTDH/LYRIC: Signaling pathways, downstream genes, interacting proteins, and regulation of tumor angiogenesis. *Advances in Cancer Research*, *120*, 75–111.

Emdad, L., Sarkar, D., Lee, S. G., Su, Z. Z., Yoo, B. K., Dash, R., et al. (2010). Astrocyte elevated gene-1: A novel target for human glioma therapy. *Molecular Cancer Therapeutics*, *9*, 79–88.

Emdad, L., Sarkar, D., Su, Z. Z., Lee, S. G., Kang, D. C., Bruce, J. N., et al. (2007). Astrocyte elevated gene-1: Recent insights into a novel gene involved in tumor progression, metastasis and neurodegeneration. *Pharmacology & Therapeutics*, *114*, 155–170.

Emdad, L., Sarkar, D., Su, Z. Z., Randolph, A., Boukerche, H., Valerie, K., et al. (2006). Activation of the nuclear factor kappaB pathway by astrocyte elevated gene-1: Implications for tumor progression and metastasis. *Cancer Research*, *66*, 1509–1516.

Engeland, C. E., Oberwinkler, H., Schumann, M., Krause, E., Muller, G. A., & Krausslich, H. G. (2011). The cellular protein lyric interacts with HIV-1 Gag. *Journal of Virology*, *85*, 13322–13332.

Erdem, H., Oktay, M., Yildirim, U., Uzunlar, A. K., & Kayikci, M. A. (2013). Expression of AEG-1 and p53 and their clinicopathological significance in malignant lesions of renal cell carcinomas: A microarray study. *Polish Journal of Pathology*, *64*, 28–32.

Erdem, H., Yildirim, U., Uzunlar, A. K., Cam, K., Tekin, A., Kayikci, M. A., et al. (2013). Relationship among expression of basic-fibroblast growth factor, MTDH/astrocyte elevated gene-1, adenomatous polyposis coli, matrix metalloproteinase 9, and COX-2 markers with prognostic factors in prostate carcinomas. *Nigerian Journal of Clinical Practice*, *16*, 418–423.

Font-Burgada, J., Sun, B., & Karin, M. (2016). Obesity and cancer: The oil that feeds the flame. *Cell Metabolism*, *23*, 48–62.

Freilinger, T., Anttila, V., de Vries, B., Malik, R., Kallela, M., Terwindt, G. M., et al. (2012). Genome-wide association analysis identifies susceptibility loci for migraine without aura. *Nature Genetics*, *44*, 777–782.

Gnosa, S., Shen, Y. M., Wang, C. J., Zhang, H., Stratmann, J., Arbman, G., et al. (2012). Expression of AEG-1 mRNA and protein in colorectal cancer patients and colon cancer cell lines. *Journal of Translational Medicine*, *10*, 109.

Gnosa, S., Zhang, H., Brodin, V. P., Carstensen, J., Adell, G., & Sun, X. F. (2014). AEG-1 expression is an independent prognostic factor in rectal cancer patients with preoperative radiotherapy: A study in a Swedish clinical trial. *British Journal of Cancer*, *111*, 166–173.

Gollavilli, P. N., Kanugula, A. K., Koyyada, R., Karnewar, S., Neeli, P. K., & Kotamraju, S. (2015). AMPK inhibits MTDH expression via GSK3beta and SIRT1 activation: Potential role in triple negative breast cancer cell proliferation. *The FEBS Journal*, *282*, 3971–3985.

Gong, Z., Liu, W., You, N., Wang, T., Wang, X., Lu, P., et al. (2012). Prognostic significance of metadherin overexpression in hepatitis B virus-related hepatocellular carcinoma. *Oncology Reports*, *27*, 2073–2079.

Gu, C., Feng, L., Peng, H., Yang, H., Feng, Z., & Yang, Y. (2015). MTDH is an oncogene in multiple myeloma, which is suppressed by Bortezomib treatment. *Oncotarget*, *7*, 4559–4569.

Guo, F., Wan, L., Zheng, A., Stanevich, V., Wei, Y., Satyshur, K. A., et al. (2014). Structural insights into the tumor-promoting function of the MTDH-SND1 complex. *Cell Reports*, *8*, 1704–1713.

Guo, J., Xia, B., Meng, F., & Lou, G. (2013). miR-137 suppresses cell growth in ovarian cancer by targeting AEG-1. *Biochemical and Biophysical Research Communications*, *441*, 357–363.

Haug, S., Schnerch, D., Halbach, S., Mastroianni, J., Dumit, V. I., Follo, M., et al. (2015). Metadherin exon 11 skipping variant enhances metastatic spread of ovarian cancer. *International Journal of Cancer*, *136*, 2328–2340.

Hayden, M. S., & Ghosh, S. (2004). Signaling to NF-kappaB. *Genes & Development*, *18*, 2195–2224.

He, J., Cao, Y., Su, T., Jiang, Y., Jiang, L., Zhou, W., et al. (2015). Downregulation of miR-375 in aldosterone-producing adenomas promotes tumour cell growth via MTDH. *Clinical Endocrinology*, *83*, 581–589.

He, X. X., Chang, Y., Meng, F. Y., Wang, M. Y., Xie, Q. H., Tang, F., et al. (2012). MicroRNA-375 targets AEG-1 in hepatocellular carcinoma and suppresses liver cancer cell growth in vitro and in vivo. *Oncogene*, *31*, 3357–3369.

He, W., He, S., Wang, Z., Shen, H., Fang, W., Zhang, Y., et al. (2015). Astrocyte elevated gene-1(AEG-1) induces epithelial-mesenchymal transition in lung cancer through activating Wnt/beta-catenin signaling. *BMC Cancer*, *15*, 107.

He, Z., He, M., Wang, C., Xu, B., Tong, L., He, J., et al. (2014). Prognostic significance of astrocyte elevated gene-1 in human astrocytomas. *International Journal of Clinical and Experimental Pathology*, *7*, 5038–5044.

Hu, G., Chong, R. A., Yang, Q., Wei, Y., Blanco, M. A., Li, F., et al. (2009). MTDH activation by 8q22 genomic gain promotes chemoresistance and metastasis of poor-prognosis breast cancer. *Cancer Cell*, *15*, 9–20.

Hu, B., Emdad, L., Bacolod, M. D., Kegelman, T. P., Shen, X. N., Alzubi, M. A., et al. (2014). Astrocyte elevated gene-1 interacts with Akt isoform 2 to control glioma growth, survival, and pathogenesis. *Cancer Research*, *74*, 7321–7332.

Hu, G., Wei, Y., & Kang, Y. (2009). The multifaceted role of MTDH/AEG-1 in cancer progression. *Clinical Cancer Research*, *15*, 5615–5620.

Huang, Y., & Li, L. P. (2014). Progress of cancer research on astrocyte elevated gene-1/metadherin (review). *Oncology Letters*, *8*, 493–501.

Huang, K., Li, L. A., Meng, Y., You, Y., Fu, X., & Song, L. (2013). High expression of astrocyte elevated gene-1 (AEG-1) is associated with progression of cervical intraepithelial neoplasia and unfavorable prognosis in cervical cancer. *World Journal of Surgical Oncology*, *11*, 297.

Huang, Y., Ren, G. P., Xu, C., Dong, S. F., Wang, Y., Gan, Y., et al. (2014). Expression of astrocyte elevated gene-1 (AEG-1) as a biomarker for aggressive pancreatic ductal adenocarcinoma. *BMC Cancer, 14,* 479.

Huang, W., Yang, L., Liang, S., Liu, D., Chen, X., Ma, Z., et al. (2013). AEG-1 is a target of perifosine and is over-expressed in gastric dysplasia and cancers. *Digestive Diseases and Sciences, 58,* 2873–2880.

Huber, O., Korn, R., McLaughlin, J., Ohsugi, M., Herrmann, B. G., & Kemler, R. (1996). Nuclear localization of beta-catenin by interaction with transcription factor LEF-1. *Mechanisms of Development, 59,* 3–10.

Isozaki, Y., Hoshino, I., Nohata, N., Kinoshita, T., Akutsu, Y., Hanari, N., et al. (2012). Identification of novel molecular targets regulated by tumor suppressive miR-375 induced by histone acetylation in esophageal squamous cell carcinoma. *International Journal of Oncology, 41,* 985–994.

Jariwala, N., Rajasekaran, D., Srivastava, J., Gredler, R., Akiel, M. A., Robertson, C. L., et al. (2015). Role of the staphylococcal nuclease and tudor domain containing 1 in oncogenesis (review). *International Journal of Oncology, 46,* 465–473.

Kang, D. C., Su, Z. Z., Sarkar, D., Emdad, L., Volsky, D. J., & Fisher, P. B. (2005). Cloning and characterization of HIV-1-inducible astrocyte elevated gene-1, AEG-1. *Gene, 353,* 8–15.

Ke, Z. F., He, S., Li, S., Luo, D., Feng, C., & Zhou, W. (2013). Expression characteristics of astrocyte elevated gene-1 (AEG-1) in tongue carcinoma and its correlation with poor prognosis. *Cancer Epidemiology, 37,* 179–185.

Khuda, I. I., Koide, N., Noman, A. S., Dagvadorj, J., Tumurkhuu, G., Naiki, Y., et al. (2009). Astrocyte elevated gene-1 (AEG-1) is induced by lipopolysaccharide as toll-like receptor 4 (TLR4) ligand and regulates TLR4 signalling. *Immunology, 128,* e700–e706.

Kim, K., Lee, S. G., Kegelman, T. P., Su, Z. Z., Das, S. K., Dash, R., et al. (2011). Role of excitatory amino acid transporter-2 (EAAT2) and glutamate in neurodegeneration: Opportunities for developing novel therapeutics. *Journal of Cellular Physiology, 226,* 2484–2493.

Kochanek, D. M., & Wells, D. G. (2013). CPEB1 regulates the expression of MTDH/AEG-1 and glioblastoma cell migration. *Molecular Cancer Research, 11,* 149–160.

Krishnan, R. K., Nolte, H., Sun, T., Kaur, H., Sreenivasan, K., Looso, M., et al. (2015). Quantitative analysis of the TNF-alpha-induced phosphoproteome reveals AEG-1/MTDH/LYRIC as an IKKbeta substrate. *Nature Communications, 6,* 6658.

Lee, S. G., Jeon, H. Y., Su, Z. Z., Richards, J. E., Vozhilla, N., Sarkar, D., et al. (2009). Astrocyte elevated gene-1 contributes to the pathogenesis of neuroblastoma. *Oncogene, 28,* 2476–2484.

Lee, H. J., Jung, D. B., Sohn, E. J., Kim, H. H., Park, M. N., Lew, J. H., et al. (2012). Inhibition of hypoxia inducible factor alpha and astrocyte-elevated gene-1 mediates cryptotanshinone exerted antitumor activity in hypoxic PC-3 cells. *Evidence-based Complementary and Alternative Medicine, 2012,* 390957.

Lee, S. G., Kang, D. C., DeSalle, R., Sarkar, D., & Fisher, P. B. (2013). AEG-1/MTDH/LYRIC, the beginning: Initial cloning, structure, expression profile, and regulation of expression. *Advances in Cancer Research, 120,* 1–38.

Lee, S. G., Kim, K., Kegelman, T. P., Dash, R., Das, S. K., Choi, J. K., et al. (2011). Oncogene AEG-1 promotes glioma-induced neurodegeneration by increasing glutamate excitotoxicity. *Cancer Research, 71,* 6514–6523.

Lee, S. G., Su, Z. Z., Emdad, L., Gupta, P., Sarkar, D., Borjabad, A., et al. (2008a). Mechanism of ceftriaxone induction of excitatory amino acid transporter-2 expression and glutamate uptake in primary human astrocytes. *The Journal of Biological Chemistry, 283,* 13116–13123.

Lee, S. G., Su, Z. Z., Emdad, L., Sarkar, D., & Fisher, P. B. (2006). Astrocyte elevated gene-1 (AEG-1) is a target gene of oncogenic Ha-ras requiring phosphatidylinositol 3-kinase and c-Myc. *Proceedings of the National Academy of Sciences of the United States of America, 103,* 17390–17395.

Lee, S. G., Su, Z. Z., Emdad, L., Sarkar, D., Franke, T. F., & Fisher, P. B. (2008b). Astrocyte elevated gene-1 activates cell survival pathways through PI3K-Akt signaling. *Oncogene, 27,* 1114–1121.

Li, C., Chen, K., Cai, J., Shi, Q. T., Li, Y., Li, L., et al. (2014). Astrocyte elevated gene-1: A novel independent prognostic biomarker for metastatic ovarian tumors. *Tumour Biology, 35,* 3079–3085.

Li, W. F., Dai, H., Ou, Q., Zuo, G. Q., & Liu, C. A. (2015). Overexpression of microRNA-30a-5p inhibits liver cancer cell proliferation and induces apoptosis by targeting MTDH/PTEN/AKT pathway. *Tumour Biology, 37,* 5885–5895.

Li, P. P., Feng, L. L., Chen, N., Ge, X. L., Lv, X., Lu, K., et al. (2015). Metadherin contributes to the pathogenesis of chronic lymphocytic leukemia partially through Wnt/beta-catenin pathway. *Medical Oncology, 32,* 479.

Li, P. P., Feng, L. L., Chen, N., Lu, K., Meng, X. H., Ge, X. L., et al. (2014). Metadherin interference inhibits proliferation and enhances chemo-sensitivity to doxorubicin in diffuse large B cell lymphoma. *International Journal of Clinical and Experimental Medicine, 7,* 2081–2086.

Li, X., Kong, X., Huo, Q., Guo, H., Yan, S., Yuan, C., et al. (2011). Metadherin enhances the invasiveness of breast cancer cells by inducing epithelial to mesenchymal transition. *Cancer Science, 102,* 1151–1157.

Li, G., Wang, Z., Ye, J., Zhang, X., Wu, H., Peng, J., et al. (2014). Uncontrolled inflammation induced by AEG-1 promotes gastric cancer and poor prognosis. *Cancer Research, 74,* 5541–5552.

Li, W. F., Wang, G., Zhao, Z. B., & Liu, C. A. (2015). High expression of metadherin correlates with malignant pathological features and poor prognostic significance in papillary thyroid carcinoma. *Clinical Endocrinology, 83,* 572–580.

Li, P. P., Yao, Q. M., Zhou, H., Feng, L. L., Ge, X. L., Lv, X., et al. (2014). Metadherin contribute to BCR signaling in chronic lymphocytic leukemia. *International Journal of Clinical and Experimental Pathology, 7,* 1588–1594.

Li, W., Zhai, L., Zhao, C., & Lv, S. (2015). MiR-153 inhibits epithelial-mesenchymal transition by targeting metadherin in human breast cancer. *Breast Cancer Research and Treatment, 150,* 501–509.

Liang, Y., Hu, J., Li, J., Liu, Y., Yu, J., Zhuang, X., et al. (2015). Epigenetic activation of TWIST1 by MTDH promotes cancer stem-like cell traits in breast cancer. *Cancer Research, 75,* 3672–3680.

Liao, W. T., Guo, L., Zhong, Y., Wu, Y. H., Li, J., & Song, L. B. (2011). Astrocyte elevated gene-1 (AEG-1) is a marker for aggressive salivary gland carcinoma. *Journal of Translational Medicine, 9,* 205.

Ligthart, L., de Vries, B., Smith, A. V., Ikram, M. A., Amin, N., Hottenga, J. J., et al. (2011). Meta-analysis of genome-wide association for migraine in six population-based European cohorts. *European Journal of Human Genetics, 19,* 901–907.

Lindskog, C., Edlund, K., Mattsson, J. S., & Micke, P. (2015). Immunohistochemistry-based prognostic biomarkers in NSCLC: Novel findings on the road to clinical use? *Expert Review of Molecular Diagnostics, 15,* 471–490.

Liu, I. J., Chiu, C. Y., Chen, Y. C., & Wu, H. C. (2011). Molecular mimicry of human endothelial cell antigen by autoantibodies to nonstructural protein 1 of dengue virus. *The Journal of Biological Chemistry, 286,* 9726–9736.

Liu, K., Guo, L., Miao, L., Bao, W., Yang, J., Li, X., et al. (2013). Ursolic acid inhibits epithelial-mesenchymal transition by suppressing the expression of astrocyte-elevated gene-1 in human nonsmall cell lung cancer A549 cells. *Anti-Cancer Drugs, 24,* 494–503.

Liu, H. Y., Liu, C. X., Han, B., Zhang, X. Y., & Sun, R. P. (2012). AEG-1 is associated with clinical outcome in neuroblastoma patients. *Cancer Biomarkers, 11,* 115–121.

Liu, Y., Su, Z., Li, G., Yu, C., Ren, S., Huang, D., et al. (2013). Increased expression of metadherin protein predicts worse disease-free and overall survival in laryngeal squamous cell carcinoma. *International Journal of Cancer, 133*, 671–679.

Liu, P., Tang, H., Chen, B., He, Z., Deng, M., Wu, M., et al. (2015). miR-26a suppresses tumour proliferation and metastasis by targeting metadherin in triple negative breast cancer. *Cancer Letters, 357*, 384–392.

Liu, L., Wu, J., Ying, Z., Chen, B., Han, A., Liang, Y., et al. (2010). Astrocyte elevated gene-1 upregulates matrix metalloproteinase-9 and induces human glioma invasion. *Cancer Research, 70*, 3750–3759.

Liu, D. C., & Yang, Z. L. (2013). MTDH and EphA7 are markers for metastasis and poor prognosis of gallbladder adenocarcinoma. *Diagnostic Cytopathology, 41*, 199–205.

Liu, X., Zhang, N., Li, X., Moran, M. S., Yuan, C., Yan, S., et al. (2011). Identification of novel variants of metadherin in breast cancer. *PloS One, 6*, e17582.

Long, M., Hao, M., Dong, K., Shen, J., Wang, X., Lin, F., et al. (2013). AEG-1 over-expression is essential for maintenance of malignant state in human AML cells via up-regulation of Akt1 mediated by AURKA activation. *Cellular Signalling, 25*, 1438–1446.

Luo, Y., Zhang, X., Tan, Z., Wu, P., Xiang, X., Dang, Y., et al. (2015). Astrocyte elevated gene-1 as a novel clinicopathological and prognostic biomarker for gastrointestinal cancers: A meta-analysis with 2999 patients. *PloS One, 10*, e0145659.

Luparello, C., Longo, A., & Vetrano, M. (2012). Exposure to cadmium chloride influences astrocyte-elevated gene-1 (AEG-1) expression in MDA-MB231 human breast cancer cells. *Biochimie, 94*, 207–213.

Lupo, J., Conti, A., Sueur, C., Coly, P. A., Coute, Y., Hunziker, W., et al. (2012). Identification of new interacting partners of the shuttling protein ubinuclein (Ubn-1). *Experimental Cell Research, 318*, 509–520.

Luxton, H. J., Barnouin, K., Kelly, G., Hanrahan, S., Totty, N., Neal, D. E., et al. (2014). Regulation of the localisation and function of the oncogene LYRIC/AEG-1 by ubiquitination at K486 and K491. *Molecular Oncology, 8*, 633–641.

Ma, J., Xie, S. L., Geng, Y. J., Jin, S., Wang, G. Y., & Lv, G. Y. (2014). In vitro regulation of hepatocellular carcinoma cell viability, apoptosis, invasion, and AEG-1 expression by LY294002. *Clinical and Research in Hepatology and Gastroenterology, 38*, 73–80.

Mangelsdorf, D. J., Ong, E. S., Dyck, J. A., & Evans, R. M. (1990). Nuclear receptor that identifies a novel retinoic acid response pathway. *Nature, 345*, 224–229.

Meng, X., Thiel, K. W., & Leslie, K. K. (2013). Drug resistance mediated by AEG-1/MTDH/LYRIC. *Advances in Cancer Research, 120*, 135–157.

Moelans, C. B., van der Groep, P., Hoefnagel, L. D., van de Vijver, M. J., Wesseling, P., Wesseling, J., et al. (2014). Genomic evolution from primary breast carcinoma to distant metastasis: Few copy number changes of breast cancer related genes. *Cancer Letters, 344*, 138–146.

Motalleb, G., Gholipour, N., & Samaei, N. M. (2014). Association of the human astrocyte elevated gene-1 promoter variants with susceptibility to hepatocellular carcinoma. *Medical Oncology, 31*, 916.

Nikpour, M., Emadi-Baygi, M., Fischer, U., Niegisch, G., Schulz, W. A., & Nikpour, P. (2014). MTDH/AEG-1 contributes to central features of the neoplastic phenotype in bladder cancer. *Urologic Oncology, 32*, 670–677.

Noch, E. K., & Khalili, K. (2013). The role of AEG-1/MTDH/LYRIC in the pathogenesis of central nervous system disease. *Advances in Cancer Research, 120*, 159–192.

Nohata, N., Hanazawa, T., Kikkawa, N., Mutallip, M., Sakurai, D., Fujimura, L., et al. (2011). Tumor suppressive microRNA-375 regulates oncogene AEG-1/MTDH in head and neck squamous cell carcinoma (HNSCC). *Journal of Human Genetics, 56*, 595–601.

Park, K. J., Yu, M. O., Song, N. H., Kong, D. S., Park, D. H., Chae, Y. S., et al. (2015). Expression of astrocyte elevated gene-1 (AEG-1) in human meningiomas and its roles in cell proliferation and survival. *Journal of Neuro-Oncology, 121,* 31–39.

Ran, C., Graae, L., Magnusson, P. K., Pedersen, N. L., Olson, L., & Belin, A. C. (2014). A replication study of GWAS findings in migraine identifies association in a Swedish case-control sample. *BMC Medical Genetics, 15,* 38.

Robertson, C. L., Srivastava, J., Rajasekaran, D., Gredler, R., Akiel, M. A., Jariwala, N., et al. (2015a). The role of AEG-1 in the development of liver cancer. *Hepatic Oncology, 2,* 303–312.

Robertson, C. L., Srivastava, J., Siddiq, A., Gredler, R., Emdad, L., Rajasekaran, D., et al. (2014). Genetic deletion of AEG-1 prevents hepatocarcinogenesis. *Cancer Research, 74,* 6184–6193.

Robertson, C. L., Srivastava, J., Siddiq, A., Gredler, R., Emdad, L., Rajasekaran, D., et al. (2015b). Astrocyte elevated gene-1 (AEG-1) regulates lipid homeostasis. *The Journal of Biological Chemistry, 290,* 18227–18236.

Rothstein, J. D., Patel, S., Regan, M. R., Haenggeli, C., Huang, Y. H., Bergles, D. E., et al. (2005). Beta-lactam antibiotics offer neuroprotection by increasing glutamate transporter expression. *Nature, 433,* 73–77.

Santarpia, M., Magri, I., Sanchez-Ronco, M., Costa, C., Molina-Vila, M. A., Gimenez-Capitan, A., et al. (2011). mRNA expression levels and genetic status of genes involved in the EGFR and NF-kappaB pathways in metastatic non-small-cell lung cancer patients. *Journal of Translational Medicine, 9,* 163.

Sarkar, D. (2013). AEG-1/MTDH/LYRIC in liver cancer. *Advances in Cancer Research, 120,* 193–221.

Sarkar, D., Emdad, L., Lee, S. G., Yoo, B. K., Su, Z. Z., & Fisher, P. B. (2009). Astrocyte elevated gene-1: Far more than just a gene regulated in astrocytes. *Cancer Research, 69,* 8529–8535.

Sarkar, D., & Fisher, P. B. (2013). AEG-1/MTDH/LYRIC: Clinical significance. *Advances in Cancer Research, 120,* 39–74.

Sarkar, D., Park, E. S., Emdad, L., Lee, S. G., Su, Z. Z., & Fisher, P. B. (2008). Molecular basis of nuclear factor-kappaB activation by astrocyte elevated gene-1. *Cancer Research, 68,* 1478–1484.

Shalapour, S., & Karin, M. (2015). Immunity, inflammation, and cancer: An eternal fight between good and evil. *The Journal of Clinical Investigation, 125,* 3347–3355.

Shen, X., Si, Y., Yang, Z., Wang, Q., Yuan, J., & Zhang, X. (2015). MicroRNA-542-3p suppresses cell growth of gastric cancer cells via targeting oncogene astrocyte-elevated gene-1. *Medical Oncology, 32,* 361.

Shi, X., & Wang, X. (2015). The role of MTDH/AEG-1 in the progression of cancer. *International Journal of Clinical and Experimental Medicine, 8,* 4795–4807.

Song, Y. H., Jeong, S. J., Kwon, H. Y., Kim, B., Kim, S. H., & Yoo, D. Y. (2012). Ursolic acid from Oldenlandia diffusa induces apoptosis via activation of caspases and phosphorylation of glycogen synthase kinase 3 beta in SK-OV-3 ovarian cancer cells. *Biological & Pharmaceutical Bulletin, 35,* 1022–1028.

Song, H., Li, C., Lu, R., Zhang, Y., & Geng, J. (2010). Expression of astrocyte elevated gene-1: A novel marker of the pathogenesis, progression, and poor prognosis for endometrial cancer. *International Journal of Gynecological Cancer, 20,* 1188–1196.

Song, L., Li, W., Zhang, H., Liao, W., Dai, T., Yu, C., et al. (2009). Over-expression of AEG-1 significantly associates with tumour aggressiveness and poor prognosis in human non-small cell lung cancer. *The Journal of Pathology, 219,* 317–326.

Srivastava, J., Robertson, C. L., Rajasekaran, D., Gredler, R., Siddiq, A., Emdad, L., et al. (2014). AEG-1 regulates retinoid X receptor and inhibits retinoid signaling. *Cancer Research, 74,* 4364–4377.

Srivastava, J., Siddiq, A., Gredler, R., Shen, X. N., Rajasekaran, D., Robertson, C. L., et al. (2015). Astrocyte elevated gene-1 and c-Myc cooperate to promote hepatocarcinogenesis in mice. *Hepatology, 61*, 915–929.

Su, Z. Z., Chen, Y., Kang, D. C., Chao, W., Simm, M., Volsky, D. J., et al. (2003). Customized rapid subtraction hybridization (RaSH) gene microarrays identify overlapping expression changes in human fetal astrocytes resulting from human immunodeficiency virus-1 infection or tumor necrosis factor-alpha treatment. *Gene, 306*, 67–78.

Su, Z. Z., Kang, D. C., Chen, Y., Pekarskaya, O., Chao, W., Volsky, D. J., et al. (2002). Identification and cloning of human astrocyte genes displaying elevated expression after infection with HIV-1 or exposure to HIV-1 envelope glycoprotein by rapid subtraction hybridization, RaSH. *Oncogene, 21*, 3592–3602.

Suh, S. S., Yoo, J. Y., Cui, R., Kaur, B., Huebner, K., Lee, T. K., et al. (2014). FHIT suppresses epithelial-mesenchymal transition (EMT) and metastasis in lung cancer through modulation of microRNAs. *PLoS Genetics, 10*, e1004652.

Sun, W., Fan, Y. Z., Xi, H., Lu, X. S., Ye, C., & Zhang, J. T. (2011). Astrocyte elevated gene-1 overexpression in human primary gallbladder carcinomas: An unfavorable and independent prognostic factor. *Oncology Reports, 26*, 1133–1142.

Sutherland, H. G., Lam, Y. W., Briers, S., Lamond, A. I., & Bickmore, W. A. (2004). 3D3/lyric: A novel transmembrane protein of the endoplasmic reticulum and nuclear envelope, which is also present in the nucleolus. *Experimental Cell Research, 294*, 94–105.

Szanto, A., Narkar, V., Shen, Q., Uray, I. P., Davies, P. J., & Nagy, L. (2004). Retinoid X receptors: X-ploring their (patho)physiological functions. *Cell Death and Differentiation, 11*(Suppl. 2), S126–S143.

Tang, Y., Liu, X., Su, B., Zhang, Z., Zeng, X., Lei, Y., et al. (2015). microRNA-22 acts as a metastasis suppressor by targeting metadherin in gastric cancer. *Molecular Medicine Reports, 11*, 454–460.

Thirkettle, H. J., Girling, J., Warren, A. Y., Mills, I. G., Sahadevan, K., Leung, H., et al. (2009). LYRIC/AEG-1 is targeted to different subcellular compartments by ubiquitinylation and intrinsic nuclear localization signals. *Clinical Cancer Research, 15*, 3003–3013.

Thirkettle, H. J., Mills, I. G., Whitaker, H. C., & Neal, D. E. (2009). Nuclear LYRIC/AEG-1 interacts with PLZF and relieves PLZF-mediated repression. *Oncogene, 28*, 3663–3670.

Tokunaga, E., Nakashima, Y., Yamashita, N., Hisamatsu, Y., Okada, S., Akiyoshi, S., et al. (2014). Overexpression of metadherin/MTDH is associated with an aggressive phenotype and a poor prognosis in invasive breast cancer. *Breast Cancer, 21*, 341–349.

Tong, L., Wang, C., Hu, X., Pang, B., Yang, Z., He, Z., et al. (2016). Correlated overexpression of metadherin and SND1 in glioma cells. *Biological Chemistry, 397*, 57–65.

Vartak-Sharma, N., Gelman, B. B., Joshi, C., Borgamann, K., & Ghorpade, A. (2014). Astrocyte elevated gene-1 is a novel modulator of HIV-1-associated neuroinflammation via regulation of nuclear factor-kappaB signaling and excitatory amino acid transporter-2 repression. *The Journal of Biological Chemistry, 289*, 19599–19612.

Vartak-Sharma, N., & Ghorpade, A. (2012). Astrocyte elevated gene-1 regulates astrocyte responses to neural injury: Implications for reactive astrogliosis and neurodegeneration. *Journal of Neuroinflammation, 9*, 195.

Wan, L., Hu, G., Wei, Y., Yuan, M., Bronson, R. T., Yang, Q., et al. (2014). Genetic ablation of metadherin inhibits autochthonous prostate cancer progression and metastasis. *Cancer Research, 74*, 5336–5347.

Wan, L., & Kang, Y. (2013). Pleiotropic roles of AEG-1/MTDH/LYRIC in breast cancer. *Advances in Cancer Research, 120*, 113–134.

Wan, L., Lu, X., Yuan, S., Wei, Y., Guo, F., Shen, M., et al. (2014). MTDH-SND1 interaction is crucial for expansion and activity of tumor-initiating cells in diverse oncogene- and carcinogen-induced mammary tumors. *Cancer Cell, 26*, 92–105.

Wang, N., Du, X., Zang, L., Song, N., Yang, T., Dong, R., et al. (2012). Prognostic impact of metadherin-SND1 interaction in colon cancer. *Molecular Biology Reports, 39*, 10497–10504.

Wang, F., Ke, Z. F., Sun, S. J., Chen, W. F., Yang, S. C., Li, S. H., et al. (2011). Oncogenic roles of astrocyte elevated gene-1 (AEG-1) in osteosarcoma progression and prognosis. *Cancer Biology & Therapy, 12*, 539–548.

Wang, F., Ke, Z. F., Wang, R., Wang, Y. F., Huang, L. L., & Wang, L. T. (2014). Astrocyte elevated gene-1 (AEG-1) promotes osteosarcoma cell invasion through the JNK/c-Jun/MMP-2 pathway. *Biochemical and Biophysical Research Communications, 452*, 933–939.

Wang, K., Lim, H. Y., Shi, S., Lee, J., Deng, S., Xie, T., et al. (2013). Genomic landscape of copy number aberrations enables the identification of oncogenic drivers in hepatocellular carcinoma. *Hepatology, 58*, 706–717.

Wang, Y. P., Liu, I. J., Chiang, C. P., & Wu, H. C. (2013a). Astrocyte elevated gene-1 is associated with metastasis in head and neck squamous cell carcinoma through p65 phosphorylation and upregulation of MMP1. *Molecular Cancer, 12*, 109.

Wang, L., Liu, Z., Ma, D., Piao, Y., Guo, F., Han, Y., et al. (2013b). SU6668 suppresses proliferation of triple negative breast cancer cells through down-regulating MTDH expression. *Cancer Cell International, 13*, 88.

Wang, B., Shen, Z. L., Jiang, K. W., Zhao, G., Wang, C. Y., Yan, Y. C., et al. (2015). MicroRNA-217 functions as a prognosis predictor and inhibits colorectal cancer cell proliferation and invasion via an AEG-1 dependent mechanism. *BMC Cancer, 15*, 437.

Wang, M., Wang, J., Deng, J., Li, X., Long, W., & Chang, Y. (2015a). MiR-145 acts as a metastasis suppressor by targeting metadherin in lung cancer. *Medical Oncology, 32*, 344.

Wang, Z., Wang, L., Hu, J., Fan, R., Zhou, J., Wang, L., et al. (2015b). RARRES3 suppressed metastasis through suppression of MTDH to regulate epithelial-mesenchymal transition in colorectal cancer. *American Journal of Cancer Research, 5*, 1988–1999.

Wang, Z., Wei, Y. B., Gao, Y. L., Yan, B., Yang, J. R., & Guo, Q. (2014). Metadherin in prostate, bladder, and kidney cancer: A systematic review. *Molecular and Clinical Oncology, 2*, 1139–1144.

Wang, Y., Wei, Y., Tong, H., Chen, L., Fan, Y., Ji, Y., et al. (2015). MiR-302c-3p suppresses invasion and proliferation of glioma cells via down-regulating metadherin (MTDH) expression. *Cancer Biology & Therapy, 16*, 1308–1315.

Ward, A., Balwierz, A., Zhang, J. D., Kublbeck, M., Pawitan, Y., Hielscher, T., et al. (2013). Re-expression of microRNA-375 reverses both tamoxifen resistance and accompanying EMT-like properties in breast cancer. *Oncogene, 32*, 1173–1182.

Wei, J., Li, Z., Chen, W., Ma, C., Zhan, F., Wu, W., et al. (2013). AEG-1 participates in TGF-beta1-induced EMT through p38 MAPK activation. *Cell Biology International, 37*, 1016–1021.

Wu, C., Jin, B., Chen, L., Zhuo, D., Zhang, Z., Gong, K., et al. (2013). MiR-30d induces apoptosis and is regulated by the Akt/FOXO pathway in renal cell carcinoma. *Cellular Signalling, 25*, 1212–1221.

Wu, H., Liu, Q., Cai, T., Chen, Y. D., Liao, F., & Wang, Z. F. (2014). MiR-136 modulates glioma cell sensitivity to temozolomide by targeting astrocyte elevated gene-1. *Diagnostic Pathology, 9*, 173.

Xia, Z., Zhang, N., Jin, H., Yu, Z., Xu, G., & Huang, Z. (2010). Clinical significance of astrocyte elevated gene-1 expression in human oligodendrogliomas. *Clinical Neurology and Neurosurgery, 112*, 413–419.

Yan, J. W., Lin, J. S., & He, X. X. (2014). The emerging role of miR-375 in cancer. *International Journal of Cancer, 135*, 1011–1018.

Yan, J. J., Zhang, Y. N., Liao, J. Z., Ke, K. P., Chang, Y., Li, P. Y., et al. (2015). MiR-497 suppresses angiogenesis and metastasis of hepatocellular carcinoma by inhibiting VEGFA and AEG-1. *Oncotarget, 6*, 29527–29542.

Yang, J., Mani, S. A., Donaher, J. L., Ramaswamy, S., Itzykson, R. A., Come, C., et al. (2004). Twist, a master regulator of morphogenesis, plays an essential role in tumor metastasis. *Cell*, *117*, 927–939.

Yang, J., Valineva, T., Hong, J., Bu, T., Yao, Z., Jensen, O. N., et al. (2007). Transcriptional co-activator protein p100 interacts with snRNP proteins and facilitates the assembly of the spliceosome. *Nucleic Acids Research*, *35*, 4485–4494.

Yang, Y., Wu, J., Guan, H., Cai, J., Fang, L., Li, J., et al. (2012). MiR-136 promotes apoptosis of glioma cells by targeting AEG-1 and Bcl-2. *FEBS Letters*, *586*, 3608–3612.

Yang, G., Zhang, L., Lin, S., Li, L., Liu, M., Chen, H., et al. (2014). AEG-1 is associated with tumor progression in nonmuscle-invasive bladder cancer. *Medical Oncology*, *31*, 986.

Yang, C., Zheng, S., Liu, Q., Liu, T., Lu, M., Dai, F., et al. (2015). Metadherin is required for the proliferation, migration, and invasion of esophageal squamous cell carcinoma and its meta-analysis. *Translational Research*, *166*, 614–626. e612.

Yin, X., Ren, M., Jiang, H., Cui, S., Wang, S., Jiang, H., et al. (2015). Downregulated AEG-1 together with inhibited PI3K/Akt pathway is associated with reduced viability of motor neurons in an ALS model. *Molecular and Cellular Neurosciences*, *68*, 303–313.

Yoo, B. K., Emdad, L., Lee, S. G., Su, Z. Z., Santhekadur, P., Chen, D., et al. (2011). Astrocyte elevated gene-1 (AEG-1): A multifunctional regulator of normal and abnormal physiology. *Pharmacology & Therapeutics*, *130*, 1–8.

Yoo, B. K., Emdad, L., Su, Z. Z., Villanueva, A., Chiang, D. Y., Mukhopadhyay, N. D., et al. (2009). Astrocyte elevated gene-1 regulates hepatocellular carcinoma development and progression. *The Journal of Clinical Investigation*, *119*, 465–477.

Yoo, B. K., Santhekadur, P. K., Gredler, R., Chen, D., Emdad, L., Bhutia, S., et al. (2011). Increased RNA-induced silencing complex (RISC) activity contributes to hepatocellular carcinoma. *Hepatology*, *53*, 1538–1548.

Zhang, B., Liu, X. X., He, J. R., Zhou, C. X., Guo, M., He, M., et al. (2011). Pathologically decreased miR-26a antagonizes apoptosis and facilitates carcinogenesis by targeting MTDH and EZH2 in breast cancer. *Carcinogenesis*, *32*, 2–9.

Zhang, N., Wang, X., Huo, Q., Sun, M., Cai, C., Liu, Z., et al. (2014). MicroRNA-30a suppresses breast tumor growth and metastasis by targeting metadherin. *Oncogene*, *33*, 3119–3128.

Zhang, F., Yang, Q., Meng, F., Shi, H., Li, H., Liang, Y., et al. (2013). Astrocyte elevated gene-1 interacts with beta-catenin and increases migration and invasion of colorectal carcinoma. *Molecular Carcinogenesis*, *52*, 603–610.

Zhao, Y., Kong, X., Li, X., Yan, S., Yuan, C., Hu, W., et al. (2011). Metadherin mediates lipopolysaccharide-induced migration and invasion of breast cancer cells. *PloS One*, *6*, e29363.

Zhao, J., Wang, W., Huang, Y., Wu, J., Chen, M., Cui, P., et al. (2014). HBx elevates oncoprotein AEG-1 expression to promote cell migration by downregulating miR-375 and miR-136 in malignant hepatocytes. *DNA and Cell Biology*, *33*, 715–722.

Zhou, C. X., Wang, C. L., Yu, A. L., Wang, Q. Y., Zhan, M. N., Tang, J., et al. (2015). MiR-630 suppresses breast cancer progression by targeting metadherin. *Oncotarget*, *7*, 1288–1299.

Zhu, H. D., Liao, J. Z., He, X. X., & Li, P. Y. (2015). The emerging role of astrocyte-elevated gene-1 in hepatocellular carcinoma (review). *Oncology Reports*, *34*, 539–546.

Zhu, K., Pan, Q., Jia, L. Q., Dai, Z., Ke, A. W., Zeng, H. Y., et al. (2014). MiR-302c inhibits tumor growth of hepatocellular carcinoma by suppressing the endothelial-mesenchymal transition of endothelial cells. *Scientific Reports*, *4*, 5524.

Zou, Y., Qin, X., Xiong, H., Zhu, F., Chen, T., & Wu, H. (2015). Apoptosis of human non-small-cell lung cancer A549 cells triggered by evodiamine through MTDH-dependent signaling pathway. *Tumour Biology*, *36*, 5187–5193.

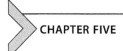

CHAPTER FIVE

Role of the RB-Interacting Proteins in Stem Cell Biology

M. Mushtaq*, H. Viñas Gaza*, E.V. Kashuba*,†,1
*Karolinska Institutet, Stockholm, Sweden
†R.E. Kavetsky Institute of Experimental Pathology, Oncology and Radiobiology, NASU, Kyiv, Ukraine
¹Corresponding author: e-mail address: elena.kashuba@ki.se

Contents

Abstract

Human retinoblastoma gene *RB1* is the first tumor suppressor gene (TSG) isolated by positional cloning in 1986. RB is extensively studied for its ability to regulate cell cycle by binding to E2F1 and inhibiting the transcriptional activity of the latter.

In human embryonic stem cells (ESCs), only a minute trace of RB is found in complex with E2F1. Increased activity of RB triggers differentiation, cell cycle arrest, and cell death. On the other hand, inactivation of the entire RB family (*RB1*, *RBL1*, and *RBL2*) in human ESC induces G_2/M arrest and cell death. These observations indicate that both loss and overactivity of RB could be lethal for the stemness of cells.

A question arises *why inactive RB is required for the survival and stemness of cells?* To shed some light on this question, we analyzed the RB-binding proteins. In this review we have focused on 27 RB-binding partners that may have potential roles in different aspects of stem cell biology.

Advances in Cancer Research, Volume 131
ISSN 0065-230X
http://dx.doi.org/10.1016/bs.acr.2016.04.002

1. INTRODUCTION

Human retinoblastoma gene *RB1* was the first tumor suppressor gene (TSG) isolated by positional cloning in 1986, and it served as prototype for identification of new TSGs (Zhu, 2005). Retinoblastoma is a sporadic or hereditary pediatric neoplasm arising from retinal cells. The cloning of *RB1* gene and identification of biallelic *RB1* mutations in retinoblastoma follow the Knudson model (1971), which states that a tumor phenotype is not apparent unless both copies of a gene are damaged (Giacinti & Giordano, 2006) (Fig. 1). Germ line mutation or deletion of *RB1* leads to heritable form of retinoblastoma in which the appearance of retinal tumors arises with an incidence of greater than 95% (Mittnacht, 2005). Importantly, *RB1* mutations have also been found in nonretinal sporadic cancers, including sarcomas, glioblastomas, small-cell lung, bladder, breast, cervical, and parathyroid cancers, supporting the notion that the gene and its encoded protein are involved in a common tumor suppressing pathway. Hereditary retinoblastoma disease is mostly a childhood malignancy with

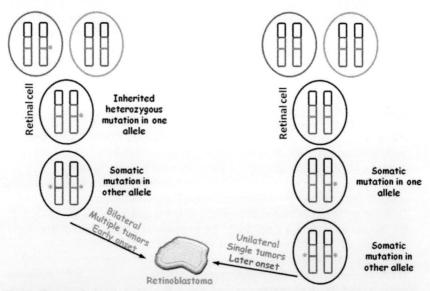

Fig. 1 The Knudson (two-hit) model showing retinoblastoma development. Germ line mutation of *RB1* leads to heritable form of retinoblastoma; bilateral retinal tumors arise often in early age (before 2 years old). This model suggests tumor initiation in sporadic form of cancer, when the second mutation must happen in specific populations of cells. These tumors are often unilateral and occur later in age (4–5 years old). * indicates mutations in *RB1* gene. (See the color plate.)

family history. The specific age window of retinoblastoma growth suggests a model of tumor initiation in which loss of RB function must happen in specific populations of cells that may be transiently present in the developing retina (Sage, 2012).

2. GENE AND PROTEIN FAMILY OF RB

RB1 gene consists of 27 exons spanning over 180 kb of genomic DNA on human chromosome 13q14. A 4.7-kb transcript encodes a nuclear phosphoprotein consisting of 928 amino acids, the retinoblastoma protein (RB/p105) (Toguchida et al., 1993). There are two RB-related proteins, RBL1/p107 and RBL2/p130, and the corresponding genes mapped to human chromosomal region 20q11.2 and 16p12.2, respectively (Giacinti & Giordano, 2006). Three RB family proteins are targeted by viral oncoproteins during viral-induced cell transformation. The common domain of RB family proteins which is specific for this binding is known as a "pocket"; hence, these three proteins are often called pocket proteins. The pocket region is structurally characterized by two conserved functional subdomains (A and B), separated by a spacer (S), which substantially differs among the three RB proteins. RBL1 and RBL2 are more related to each other, showing about 50% amino acid identity, while similarity to RB is lower (30–35% identity). Interestingly, mutations in *RBL1* and *RBL2* are extremely rare in human cancers (Goodrich, 2006).

3. MOLECULAR DETAILS OF RB FUNCTION

RB is extensively studied for its ability to regulate the cell cycle by binding to E2F1 and inhibiting the transcriptional activity of the latter. Interaction of RB and E2F1 is controlled through phosphorylation of RB by cyclin-dependent kinases (CDKs) (Sherr, 1993). RB in its unphosphorylated form binds and inactivates E2F1; phosphorylated RB cannot interact with E2F1. The growth factors-dependent CDKs— CDK4 and CDK6 operate during the first 80–90% of G1 phase, while growth signal-independent CDKs—CDK1, CDK2, and CDK3 are active in the rest of cell cycle (Hunter & Pines, 1994; Weinberg, 2007). At different stages of the cell cycle CDKs need cyclin molecules, namely, Cyclin D, Cyclin E, and Cyclin A (Fig. 2, left panel) as a guide for phosphorylation of RB (Morgan, 1995). Apart from cyclins, cells also deploy CDK inhibitors that bind to CDKs and inhibit phosphorylation of RB (Hirama & Koeffler,

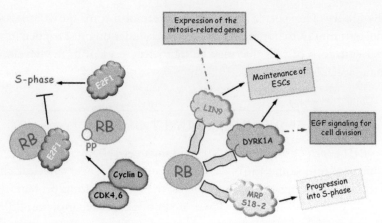

Fig. 2 RB controls induction of S-phase of cell cycle. *Left panel*: RB when unphosphorylated binds to E2F1, inactivating the transcriptional activity of the latter. Phosphorylated RB does not bind the E2F1, and S-phase entry is induced. CDKs together with cyclins phosphorylate the RB. *Right panel*: Inhibitory effect of binding between RB and E2F1 on cell cycle regulation is limited in stem cells. RB is involved in control of SCs cell cycle through binding with LIN9, DYRK1A, and S18-2 proteins. *Blue* shapes (*wavy*) show binding between RB and discussed proteins. (See the color plate.)

1995). CDK inhibitors are classified into two categories: (i) inhibitors of CK4/6—CDKN2A, CDKN2B, CDKN2C, and CDKN2D; (ii) CDK1, 2, and 3 inhibitors—CDKN1A, CDKN1B, and CDKN1C (Schwaller et al., 1997). RB inactivation leads to uncontrolled cell division that might result in development of cancer. Cancerogenesis is an evolutionary process, based on adaptation of different mechanisms for RB inactivation, including mutations, deletions, epigenetic silencing of *RB1* promoter, inactivation of CDK inhibitors, mutation in *CDK* genes, and recruitment of certain proteins that bind RB and prevent its association to E2F1 (Weinberg, 2007).

It has been suggested that a small pool of active RB is required for the maintenance of stem cells (SCs). In human embryonic stem cells (ESCs), RB is present mainly in hypophosphorylated and hyperphosphorylated states, and only minute traces of RB are found in complex with E2F1 (Conklin, Baker, & Sage, 2012). Moreover, increased activity of RB triggers differentiation, cell cycle arrest, and cell death. On the other hand, inactivation of the entire RB family (*RB1*, *RBL1*, and *RBL2*) in human ESC induces G_2/M arrest and cell death through functional activation of the p53 pathway, ie, induction of CDKN1A (Conklin et al., 2012). These observations indicate that both loss and overactivity of RB could be lethal for the stemness of SCs.

A question arises why inactive RB is required for the survival and stemness of cells? To answer the question, we analyzed the RB-binding proteins. In this review we have focused on those RB-binding partners that may have potential roles in different aspects of stem cell biology (Tables 1 and S1 (http://dx.doi.org/10.1016/bs.acr.2016.04.002)). All proteins discussed in this chapter are listed in Table 2.

Table 1 RB-Interacting Proteins Involved in Control on Cell Stemness and Differentiation

No	Protein Acronym	Protein Name	Accession Number at NCBI	Synonyms
1	CEBPA	CCAAT/enhancer-binding protein, alpha	NP_001272758	C/EBP-ALPHA, CEBP
2	CEBPB	CCAAT/enhancer-binding protein, beta	NP_001272807	IL6DBP, LAP, NFIL6, TCF5
3	CENPF	Centromeric protein F	NP_057427	LEK1
4	DNMT1	DNA methyltransferase 1	NP_001124295	MCMT, CXXC9, DNMT
5	DYRK1A	Dual-specificity tyrosine phosphorylation-regulated kinase 1A	NP_001387	DYRK, MNBH
6	EID1	CREBBP/EP300 inhibitory protein 1	NP_055150	CRI1, C15ORF3
7	HBP1	HMG box-containing protein 1	NP_001231191	FLJ16340
8	HDAC1	Histone deacetylase 1	NP_004955	–
9	KDM5A	Lysine-specific demethylase 5A	NP_001036068	JARID1A, RBBP2
10	LDB1	LIM domain-binding 1	NP_001106878	CLIM2, NL1
11	LIN9	*C. elegans*, homolog of Lin9	NP_001257338	LIN9
12	LMO2	LIM domain only 2	NP_001135787	RBTN2, RHOM2, TTG2
13	MRPS18B	Mitochondrial ribosomal protein S18B	NP_054765	MRPS18-2
14	MYOD1	Myogenic differentiation antigen 1	NP_002469	MYOD, MYF3

Continued

Table 1 RB-Interacting Proteins Involved in Control on Cell Stemness and Differentiation—cont'd

No	Protein Acronym	Protein Name	Accession Number at NCBI	Synonyms
15	PELP1	Proline-, glutamic acid-, and leucine-rich protein 1	NP_001265170	MNAR
16	PHB	Prohibitin	NP_002625	–
17	PSMD10	Proteasome 26S subunit, non-ATPase, 10	NP_002805	p28, Gankyrin
18	RING1	Ring finger protein 1	NP_002922	RING1A, RNF1
19	SIN3A	SIN3 transcription regulator family member A	NP_001138829	–
20	SIRT1	Sirtuin 1	NP_001135970	SIR2L1, SIR2-ALPHA
21	SKI	V-Ski avian sarcoma viral oncogene homolog	NP_003027	SK
22	SMARCA4	SWI/SNF-related, matrix-associated, actin-dependent regulator of chromatin, subfamily A, member 4	NP_001122316	BRG1
23	TAL1	T-cell acute lymphocytic leukemia 1	NP_001274276	SCL, TCL5
24	TCF3	Transcription factor 3	NP_001129611	E2A, ITF1, VDIR
25	TRAP1	Tumor necrosis factor receptor-associated protein 1	NP_001258978	HSP75, HSP90L
26	UHRF2	Ubiquitin-like protein containing PHD and ring finger domains 2	NP_690856	NIRF, E3 ubiquitin protein ligase
27	ZBTB7A	Zinc finger- and BTB domain-containing protein 7A	NP_001304919	FBI1, LRF, POKEMON

Table 2 A List of Proteins Discussed in this Chapter

No	Protein Acronym	Protein Name	Accession Number at NCBI	Synonyms
1	ALPL	Alkaline phosphatase, liver	NP_001274101	TNSALP, TNAP
2	BGLAP	Bone gamma-carboxyglutamic acid protein	NP_001292377	BGP, osteocalcin (OC)
3	BMP1	Bone morphogenetic protein 1	NP_001190	TLD, procollagen C-proteinase
4	CCNA	Cyclin A	NP_001228	–
5	CCND1	Cyclin D1	NP_444284	PRAD1, BCL1
6	CCNE1	Cyclin E1	NP_001229	–
7	CDK1	Cyclin-dependent kinase 1	NP_001163877	CDC2, p34
8	CDK2	Cyclin-dependent kinase 2	NP_001277159	p33
9	CDK3	Cyclin-dependent kinase 3	NP_001249	–
10	CDK4	Cyclin-dependent kinase 4	NP_000066	PSK-J3, CMM3
11	CDK6	Cyclin-dependent kinase 6	NP_001138778	PLSTIRE
12	CDKN1A	Cyclin-dependent kinase inhibitor 1A	NP_000380	p21, WAF1, CIP1
13	CDKN1B	Cyclin-dependent kinase inhibitor 1B	NP_004055	KIP1, p27
14	CDKN1C	Cyclin-dependent kinase inhibitor 1C	NP_000067	KIP2, p57
15	CDKN2A	Cyclin-dependent kinase inhibitor 2A	NP_000068	p16, INK4A, INK4, CDKN2
16	CDKN2B	Cyclin-dependent kinase inhibitor 2B	NP_004927	p15, INK4B, MTS2, TP15, CDK4B INHIBITOR
17	CDKN2C	Cyclin-dependent kinase inhibitor 2C	NP_001253	p18, INK4C
18	CDKN2D	Cyclin-dependent kinase inhibitor 2D	NP_001791	p19, INK4D
19	CREBBP	CREB-binding protein	NP_001073315	CBP
20	CTNNB1	Catenin, beta-1	NP_001091679	Cadherin-associated protein, beta
21	DLL4	Delta-like 4	NP_061947	–
22	E2F1	E2F transcription factor 1	NP_005216	RBP3, RBAP1

Continued

Table 2 A List of Proteins Discussed in this Chapter—cont'd

No	Protein Acronym	Protein Name	Accession Number at NCBI	Synonyms
23	EGFR	Epidermal growth factor receptor	NP_005219	ERBB, V-ERB-B, ERBB1, HER1, SA7
24	ELF1	E74-like factor 1	NP_001138825	ETS-related transcription factor
25	FUT4	Fucosyltransferase 4	NP_002024	LeX, CD15, ELFT, FCT3A, FUTIV, SSEA-1, FUC-TIV
26	GATA1	GATA-binding protein 1	NP_002040	ERYF1, GF1
27	INHBA	Inhibin, beta-A	NP_002183	Activin A, FRP, EDF
28	KLF4	Kruppel-like factor 4	NP_004226	EZF,GKLF
29	MXI1	Max-interacting protein 1	NP_001008541	–
30	MYC	V-MYC avian myelocytomatosis viral oncogene homolog	NP_002458	–
31	NANOG	Homeobox transcription factor Nanog	NP_001284627	FLJ12581
32	NKX2-5	Nk2 homeobox 5	NP_001159647	NKX2E, CSX1, CSX
33	OPA1	Dynamin-like 120-KDa protein, mitochondrial	NP_056375	KIAA0567
34	POU5F1	POU domain, class 5, transcription factor 1	NP_001167002	OCT4, OTF4, OTF3/OCT3
35	PROM1	Prominin 1	NP_001139319	PROML1, CD133, AC133
36	RB	Retinoblastoma 1	NP_000312	p105, RB1
37	RBL1	Retinoblastoma-like 1	NP_002886	p107, CP107, p107
38	RBL2	Retinoblastoma-like 2	NP_005602	RB2, p130
39	RNF2	Ring finger protein 2	NP_009143	RING2, RING1B, HIPI3, DING, BAP1
40	SMARCA2	SWI/SNF-related, matrix-associated, actin-dependent regulator of chromatin, subfamily A, member 2	NP_001276325	SNF2L2, BRM

Table 2 A List of Proteins Discussed in this Chapter—cont'd

No	Protein Acronym	Protein Name	Accession Number at NCBI	Synonyms
41	SOX2	SRY-Box 2	NP_003097	–
42	SPI1	Spleen focus forming virus proviral integration oncogene	NP_001074016	PU.1
43	SPRY2	Sprouty *Drosophila* homolog of 2	NP_005833	–
44	TGFB1	Transforming growth factor, beta-1	NP_000651	TGFB, TGF-BETA
45	UHRF1	Ubiquitin-like protein containing PHD and ring finger domains 1	NP_001041666	ICBP90, NP95
46	VEGFA	Vascular endothelial growth factor A	NP_001020537	VEGF
47	ZFP42	Zinc finger protein 42	NP_001291287	REX1

4. INHIBITORY EFFECT OF BINDING BETWEEN RB AND E2F1 ON CELL CYCLE REGULATION IS LIMITED IN STEM CELLS

SCs have an abbreviated cell cycle with very short G_1 phase compared with differentiating cells, ie, 2–3 h vs 12–15 h (Becker et al., 2006). It was reported that RB binds DYRK1A (dual-specificity tyrosine phosphorylation-regulated kinase 1A) (Varjosalo et al., 2013). In the progeny of dividing neural stem cells (NSCs), DYRK1A participates in the regulation of EGFR (epidermal growth factor receptor) signaling. When DRYK1A is expressed at normal levels, the endocytosis–mediated degradation of EGFR is blocked. Such mechanism of EGFR degradation requires the presence of phosphorylated SPRY2 (sprouty homolog 2) protein, another modulator of EGFR signaling. It was found that deletion of *DYRK1A* in NSCs results in defective self-renewal, EGF-dependent cell fate commitment and long-term in vivo survival (Ferron et al., 2010).

Earlier we have shown that binding between RB and E2F1 might be disrupted by mitochondrial ribosomal protein S18-2 (MRPS18-2, S18-2 later in the text) that compete E2F1 to interact with RB. Noteworthy, S18-2 can bind both forms of RB, phosphorylated and unphosphorylated.

Furthermore, ectopically expressed S18-2 in rat embryonic fibroblast (REF) disrupts the cell cycle distribution, leading to immortalization of REF. Upon overexpression of S18-2, high levels of free E2F1 were observed in the nucleus and consequently, an advancement of G_1 to S phase of the cell cycle (Kashuba et al., 2008, 2009).

It was reported that LIN9 is a RB-binding protein (Gagrica et al., 2004). LIN9 is a subunit of DREAM (dimerization partner, RB-like, E2F, and multivulval class B) complex. DREAM is a multiprotein complex, which is required for the maintenance of inner cell mass and early development in embryos. The function of the DREAM complex is to regulate the cell cycle by repressing gene expression during quiescence (G_0). One of the target genes of DREAM is *CMYC*. LIN9 knockdown disrupted the cell cycle distribution in ESCs and led to accumulation of cells in G_2 and M phase, resulting in a rise in number of polyploid cells. Genome-wide expression studies showed that *LIN9* diminishing at mRNA level resulted in down-regulation of mitotic genes and an increase of differentiation-related genes. Mitotic genes are the direct targets of LIN9, as revealed by ChIP-on-chip experiments. Importantly, LIN9 deficiency did not influence the expression level of pluripotency markers, namely, SOX2 (SRY-Box 2), POU5F1 (POU domain class 5 transcription factor 1, or OCT4), and NANOG. Moreover, ESCs with depleted *LIN9* retained ALPL (alkaline phosphatase liver) activity. These studies indicate that LIN9 is significant for the proliferation and genome stability of ESCs by activating mitosis and cytokinesis-related important genes (Esterlechner et al., 2013). A summarizing schema on these interactions is shown in Fig. 2.

5. RB-INTERACTING PROTEINS ARE INVOLVED IN MAINTENANCE OF PLURIPOTENCY AND SELF-RENEWAL OF STEM CELLS

Pluripotent SCs have the potential to differentiate into any type of cells in the body. In developing embryos, approximately 96 h after fertilization, the totipotent cells start to form a cluster of cells, known as a blastocyst. In the blastocyst, a proportion of cells (known as the inner cell mass) are the pluripotent stem cells that will differentiate to create the cells and tissues of the body. All adult tissues have a certain population of multipotent SCs that differentiate in case of depletion of cells in that organ. Therefore, a balance between the self-renewal and differentiation of SCs is tightly controlled.

Apart from the control of lineage-specific differentiation of SCs, RB has been found to interact with several proteins that are important for the maintenance of pluripotency of SCs.

It was reported that EID1 (CREBBP/EP300 inhibitory protein 1) binds to the LXCXE-binding motif of RB1 (MacLellan, Xiao, Abdellatif, & Schneider, 2000). EID1 functions as transcriptional activator in association with CBP (CREB-binding protein). In protein complex with NANOG the heterodimer CBP/EID1 is recruited to the NANOG-binding DNA loci. This facilitates the formation of the long-range chromatin looping structures, which are important for the maintenance of ESC-specific gene expression. Further functional studies demonstrated that looping structures formed as a result of EID1/CBP binding contain enhancer activities. Probably, it is needed for agglomeration of the factors for transcriptional activation of genes that are involved in pluripotency and self-renewal (Fang et al., 2014) (see Fig. 3).

We have shown that the expression of stem cell markers *SOX2*, *OCT4*, *FUT4* (producing SSEA1), and *KLF4* (Kruppel-like factor 4) was induced in REFs, immortalized by overexpression of S18-2. Moreover, immortalized cells showed enhanced expression of cytochrome C oxidase*s*, NADH dehydrogenases, superoxide dismutase, ATP synthases, glutathione peroxidases that are the characteristic of highly proliferating cells (Kashuba et al., 2009; Yenamandra et al., 2012).

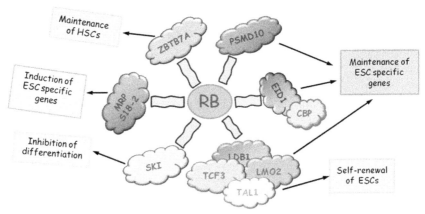

Fig. 3 RB is involved in maintenance of pluripotency of stem cells. RB-interacting proteins are involved in control on expression of genes that are implicated in maintenance of pluripotency and self-renewal of stem cells. *Blue* shapes (*wavy*) show binding between RB and discussed proteins. (See the color plate.)

Interestingly, RB forms a pentamer complex with LDB1 protein (LIM domain-binding 1) along with three other proteins—TCF3 (transcription factor 3), LMO2 (LIM domain only 2), and TAL1 (T–cell acute lymphocytic leukemia 1) (Vitelli et al., 2000). It was shown that LDB1 protein is involved in the maintenance of hematopoietic stem cells (HSCs) (Welinder & Murre, 2011). This protein binds with the non–DNA-binding adaptor protein, the LMO2 and transcription factors TCF3, TAL1, and GATA-1 in hematopoietic lineage cells (Li et al., 2011).

TCF3 plays an essential role in self-renewal of mouse ESC, as suggested by the fact that the protein complex of TCF3, OCT4, SOX2, and NANOG is formed on chromatin. Both protein complexes, TCF3-β-catenin and TCF1-β-catenin, contribute to WNT-mediated induction of SCs-related gene signature and self-renewal. Noteworthy, it was shown that combinations of TCF3 and TCF1 recruit the WNT stabilized β-catenin to the binding sites of OCT4 to the chromatin in ESCs (Yi et al., 2011) (Fig. 3).

LMO2 protein consists of two LIM domains, each comprised of zinc-finger-like tandem structures. LIM domain functions as a platform for the protein–protein binding. LIM domain of LMO2 interacts with TAL1, GATA1, LDB1, and TCF3 basic helix–loop–helix (bHLH) proteins, forming a DNA-binding complex, as discussed earlier. This multiprotein complex is capable to bind the DNA through Zn fingers of GATA1 and the bHLH motifs of TAL1 and TCF3 (Nam & Rabbitts, 2006). Of note, mice with homozygous mutations of *LMO2* failed in erythropoiesis (in yolk sac), and embryonic lethality was observed around E10.5 (Warren et al., 1994). Moreover, in vitro erythroid differentiation was inhibited in yolk sac tissue obtained from *LMO2* null mutant mice and also in double-mutant ESCs with sequentially targeted *LMO2*. Similar effects were observed in Xenopus and zebrafish embryos, LMO2 protein has a synergistic role in erythropoiesis, by forming a complex with TAL1 and GATA1 (Gering, Yamada, Rabbitts, & Patient, 2003; Mead, Deconinck, Huber, Orkin, & Zon, 2001). As described earlier, LMO2 contributes to the pluripotency of SCs also through binding with LDB1 protein (Li et al., 2011).

RB can bind directly to SKI (Tokitou et al., 1999), a transcriptional corepressor that inhibits the expression of target genes downstream of the TGF-β (transforming growth factor-β) superfamily (Deheuninck & Luo, 2009). This protein family includes TGF-β, BMP (bone morphogenetic protein), and Inhibin β-A. SKI does not possess the ability to directly bind the DNA (Nicol & Stavnezer, 1998), but binds to the active form of SMAD complexes instead, inhibiting their ability to initiate gene expression. The SMAD signaling circuit is closely linked to HSC regulation (Blank et al., 2006; Singbrant et al., 2014), suggesting that SKI may play a regulatory role in hematopoiesis. The overexpression of SKI-induced HSCs and expression of genes associated with myeloid differentiation. In hematopoiesis, SKI is independent of its ability to suppress TGF-β signaling. However, the function of SKI is partially dependent on signaling pathway induced by hepatocyte growth factor in myeloid progenitor cells (Singbrant et al., 2014) (see Fig. 3).

ZBTB7A protein (zinc finger- and BTB domain containing protein 7A) binds to SP1-binding site located at the *RB1* promoter region (Jeon et al., 2008). ZBTB7A can stabilize the pluripotency of HSCs, acting as an erythroid-specific repressor of DLL4 protein (delta-like 4). *ZBTB7A* deletion in erythroblasts caused upregulation of DLL4, sensitizing HSCs to T-cell instructive signals in the bone marrow (Lee et al., 2013). DLL4 serves as a ligand for NOTCH receptor and the NOTCH signaling regulates the fate of lymphoid lineage. It is also important for the development of hematopoiesis in mouse embryos (Yan et al., 2001) (see Fig. 3).

It was shown that PSMD10 (proteasome 26S subunit non-ATPase 10) binds to RB through fifth ankyrin repeat (Li & Tsai, 2002). Interestingly, expression of Prominin 1, a cancer SCs marker, was tightly correlated with PSMD10 expression in colorectal carcinoma. Knocking down of *PSMD10* resulted in decreased expression of VEGFA (vascular endothelial growth factor A) and stemness factors, namely, NANOG and OCT4. Expression of PSMD10 and those stemness factors discussed earlier was significantly higher in adenomas, than in the surrounding normal mucosa. Importantly, a direct correlation was observed between the expression of *PSMD10*, *VEGFA*, *NANOG*, and stages of colorectal adenomas (Mine et al., 2013).

6. RB BY INTERACTING WITH DIFFERENTIATION-RELATED FACTORS GOVERNS THE LINEAGE SPECIFICATION OF STEM CELLS

RB protein is involved in the regulation of myogenesis, cardiogenesis, and adipogenesis. RB performs a strict control of lineage commitment and differentiation of adipocytes; it determines the switch between brown and white adipocytes. RB pathway also modulates the cell commitment and differentiation of hematopoietic progenitor cells (Galderisi, Cipollaro, & Giordano, 2006).

CEBPA (CCAAT/enhancer-binding protein-alpha) binds the hypophosphorylated form of RB (Chen, Riley, Chen-Kiang, & Lee, 1996). 3T3 cells isolated from *RBL1/RBL2* knockout mice expressed endogenous CEBPA, so upon stimulation they differentiated to adipocytes. In contrast, the 3T3 cells isolated from *RB1* knockout mice did not express CEBPA; therefore, they could not differentiate in vitro into adipocyte. Moreover, the ectopic expression of RB in wild-type 3T3 promoted differentiation, while RBL1 overexpression did not induce adipogenesis (Classon, Kennedy, Mulloy, & Harlow, 2000).

RB contributes also to hematopoietic cell lineage and maturation through interaction with several hematopoietic transcription factors, such as CEBPB (CEBP-beta), SPI1 (spleen focus forming virus proviral integration oncogene), and ELF1 (E74-like factor 1) (Bergh, Ehinger, Olsson, Jacobsen, & Gullberg, 1999). RB can define the choice between monocytic and neutrophilic commitment of the CD34+ pluripotent cells. Monocyte maturation is correlated with an increased level of hypophosphorylated RB (Bergh et al., 1999). Monocyte differentiation was diverted to neutrophilic differentiation, when *RB1* was knocked out in bone marrow progenitor cells, following the treatment with cytokines promoting monocytic differentiation. RB might play dual role in lineage specification; it binds to CEBPB and induces monocyte differentiation at the same time it inhibits the activation of neutrophilic-specific transcription factors (Bergh et al., 1999).

RB interacts with the bHLH motif of MYOD1 (myogenic differentiation antigen 1) (Gu et al., 1993). This cooperation induces the activation of muscle-specific gene expression (Novitch, Mulligan, Jacks, & Lassar, 1996). Overexpression of MYOD1 in *RB1* depleted primary mouse fibroblasts induces abnormal muscle differentiation with the lack of late skeletal differentiation markers. RB effects the early phases of myogenesis in satellite myoblasts, the pool of SCs in postnatal skeletal muscles.

RB1 knockout cells showed delay in the expression of cardiac-specific transcription factors and consequently, in the entire process of cardiac differentiation. The phenotypical changes of cardiomyocytes derived from $RB1^{-/-}$ ESCs were restored by reintroducing RB in cardiac progenitors, by ectopic expression of Homeobox protein Nkx2.5 or by stimulating the BMP-dependent cardiogenic pathway. CENPF (centromeric protein F) can bind with all three pocket proteins—RBL1, RBL2, and RB (Ashe, Pabon-Pena, Dees, Price, & Bader, 2004). CENPF depletion or specific interruption of RB—CENPF interaction in the nucleus of differentiating ESCs recapitulated the delay in cardiac differentiation of *RB1* knockout ESC.

RB protein can also bind HBP1 (HMG box-containing protein 1), a transcriptional repressor (Lavender, Vandel, Bannister, & Kouzarides, 1997). HBP1 is an important regulator of neurogenesis, since it is upregulated during neurogenic stages (E13.5–E15.5) of mouse embryogenesis. HBP1 protein acts as a cell cycle inhibitor by suppressing downstream target genes of the WNT signaling and cell cycle-related genes, including *c-jun*, *cyclin D1*, *CDKN1A*, and *N-MYC* (Watanabe, Kageyama, & Ohtsuka, 2015).

Another RB-binding protein, PELP1 (proline-, glutamic acid-, and leucine-rich protein 1), is temporally expressed during the proliferation and osteogenic differentiation of rat bone marrow mesenchymal stem cells (rBMSCs) (Balasenthil & Vadlamudi, 2003). In osteogenic cultures, expression of *PELP1* at mRNA level was similar to the *BGLAP* (bone gamma–carboxyglutamic acid protein) expression, an osteogenic marker. The proliferation of undifferentiated rBMSCs was prevented by *PELP1* depletion, and bone markers BGP and ALPL were downregulated in rBMSCs cultured in routine and osteogenic differentiation media (Wang et al., 2013) (summarized in Fig. 4).

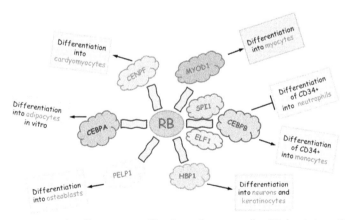

Fig. 4 RB governs the lineage specification of stem cells. RB by interacting with differentiation-related factors controls the lineage specification and differentiation of a subset of stem cells. *Blue* shapes (*wavy*) show binding between RB and discussed proteins. (See the color plate.)

7. EPIGENETIC REGULATION OF EXPRESSION OF SC-SPECIFIC GENES BY RB-BINDING PROTEINS

During mammalian development and ESC differentiation, the genome undergoes major epigenetic alterations. For example, SCs giving rise to skeletal muscle switch from fatty acid oxidation to glycolysis during the transition from quiescence to proliferation. This reprogramming of cellular metabolism decreases intracellular NAD^+ and lower activity of the histone deacetylase SIRT1 (sirtuin 1). E2F1 protein mediates the interaction between SIRT1 and RB, as shown for mouse cells (Wang et al., 2006). The diminished activity of SIRT1 resulted in increased acetylation of the H4K16 residue and activation of transcription of muscle-specific genes. Selective genetic ablation of the SIRT1 deacetylase domain in skeletal muscle results in elevated H4K16 acetylation and deregulated activation of myogensis in SCs. Moreover, mice with muscle-specific inactivation of the SIRT1 deacetylase domain exhibited defective muscle regeneration, decreased myofiber size, and de-repression of muscle developmental genes (Ryall et al., 2015).

RB interacts also with DNMT1 (DNA methyltransferase 1) and modulates its activity (Pradhan & Kim, 2002). The DNMT1 upholds methylation patterns of parental cell on daughter DNA strands during mitosis. However, the precise role of DNMT1 in regulation of quiescent adult SCs is not known. DNMT1-deficient HSCs displayed lower self-renewal, impaired niche retention, and they lost the ability to differentiate into multilineage hematopoietic cells. DNMT1 regulates distinct patterns of methylation and expression of discrete gene families in HSCs, multipotent and also the tissue-specific progenitor cells, indicating that DNMT1 differentially controls these populations of cells (Trowbridge, Snow, Kim, & Orkin, 2009).

KMD5A (lysine-specific demethylase 5A) binds RB, RBL1l and RBL2 but with different specificities (Kim, Otterson, Kratzke, Coxon, & Kaye, 1994). KMD5A functions as H3K4 demethylase (Klose et al., 2007). It was shown that KMD5A epigenetically silences several genes, involved in differentiation of SCs. Noteworthy, RB binds to KMD5A and activates repressed genes required for differentiation. KMD5A and RB colocalize in the nucleus, and RB-RBP2 complexes were detected in chromatin isolated from differentiating cells (Benevolenskaya, Murray, Branton, Young, & Kaelin, 2005).

The ubiquitin ligase UHRF2 (ubiquitin-like protein containing PHD and ring finger domains 2) induces G_1 cell cycle arrest by interacting with multiple cell cycle-related proteins, including cyclins (A2, B1, D1, and E1), p53, and RB (Mori, Ikeda, Fukushima, Takenoshita, & Kochi, 2011). UHRF2, similar to UHRF1 is an essential cofactor for the maintenance of DNA methylation. UHRF1 is expressed predominantly in pluripotent SCs, while UHRF2 is upregulated during differentiation and highly expressed in differentiated tissues. Overexpression of UHRF2 in *UHRF1* knockout ESCs did not restore DNA methylation at major satellites, indicating functional differences between them. It was proposed that the cooperative interplay of UHRF2 domains lead to a strict epigenetic control of gene expression in differentiated cells (Pichler et al., 2011).

RB physically interacts with HDAC proteins through the pocket domain (Brehm et al., 1998). It is known that the 18 genes code for histone deacetylases in the mammalian genomes, forming four groups. In spite of resemblances in their enzymatic activities, each individual member of the HDAC protein family performs a highly specific function during development and differentiation. HDAC inhibitors are of interest since under defined conditions they have potential to promote either self-renewal or differentiation of ESCs. In addition, HDAC inhibitors can induce directed differentiation of embryonic and lineage-restricted SCs toward the neuronal, cardiomyocytic, and hepatic cells (Kretsovali, Hadjimichael, & Charmpilas, 2012).

Ring finger proteins (RING1 and RNF2) are essential member of polycomb repressive complex 1 (PRC1). RB binds to RING1 and acts as modulator for the ubiquitin E3 ligase activity of RNF2 toward histone H2A at lysine 119 (summarized in Fig. 5). RING1/RNF2 preserves the ESCs identity, repressing epigenetically the transcription of developmental regulators (for mouse). A significant proportion of the PRC1 target genes are also repressed by OCT4. The recruitment of PRC1 at promoters of the target genes is OCT4 dependent, whereas engagement of OCT4 is PRC1 independent (Endoh et al., 2008). *RNF2* deficiency causes gastrulation arrest and cell cycle inhibition (Voncken et al., 2003). The loss of *RNF2* results in aberrant expression of the key developmental genes and impaired regulation of differentiation-related pathways, including TGF-β signaling, cell cycle regulation, and cellular communication. Moreover, ESC markers, including ZFP42 (zinc finger protein 42) and SOX2, were also downregulated following the depletion of RNF2 (van der Stoop et al., 2008).

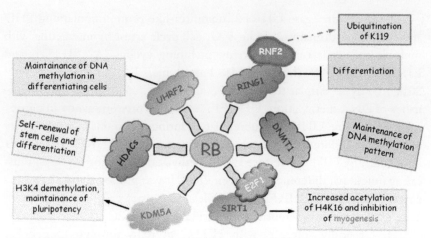

Fig. 5 RB interferes with epigenetic regulation of SC-specific genes. RB binds to proteins representing histone deacetylases, methyltransferases, demethylases, and ubiquitin ligases. This leads to finely tuned expression of SC-specific genes. *Blue* shapes (*wavy*) show binding between RB and discussed proteins. (See the color plate.)

8. RB-ASSOCIATED PROTEINS ARE INVOLVED IN STEM CELLS-DEPENDENT TISSUE HOMEOSTASIS

In a complex tissue environment a tight regulation of cell number is achieved by different physiological processes. Apoptosis, proliferation, SCs differentiation maintenance of pluripotency, and cell cycle quiescence are examples of mechanisms adopted by different cells within a tissue to stabilize homeostasis. Deregulation of any of the homeostatic mechanisms leads to serious disease conditions. SCs contribute to tissue homeostasis during the whole life span of eukaryotic organisms. In principle, SCs must have a molecular mechanism that prevents senescence by suppressing the main senescence-related pathways, which are the CDKN2A-RB pathway, p14ARF-p53 pathway, and also regulation of telomere length.

PHB (prohibitin) physically interacts with all three RB family proteins (Wang, Nath, Adlam, & Chellappan, 1999). PHB is a nuclear tumor suppressor protein that regulates the expression of p53 upon apoptotic stimuli. In response to stress, PHB is transported from the nucleus to cytoplasm and to mitochondria. PHB is highly expressed in undifferentiated ESCs, but during differentiation its expression was reduced. Deficiency of *PHB* triggered apoptosis in pluripotent ESCs, whereas ectopic expression of PHB enhanced the proliferation of ESCs. However, elevated expression of PHB blocked

ESCs differentiation into endodermal and neuronal cells. Overexpression of PHB increased the processing of OPA1 (dynamin–like 120-KDa mitochondrial protein), a GTPase controlling cristae remodeling, and mitochondrial fusion (Kowno et al., 2014).

It was reported that RB binds to SMARCA4 (SWI/SNF-related, matrix-associated, actin-dependent regulator of chromatin, subfamily A, member 4) and induces cell cycle arrest (Dunaief et al., 1994). SMARCA4 is a chromatin remodeling factor which is critical for the maintenance of SCs population in a tissue-specific manner (Corsini et al., 2009). Pan-epithelial deletion of *SMARCA4* in the small intestine resulted in crypt ablation, while partial deficiency of *SMARCA4* led to gradual repopulation of wild-type cells in the intestinal mucosa. On the other hand, *SMARCA4* deficiency in the large intestinal epithelium was compensated by upregulation of SMARCA2. Therefore, it was suggested that SMARCA4 is necessary for the survival and function of progenitor and differentiated cells in intestinal epithelium (Holik et al., 2013).

We have shown that S18-2 could enhance the telomerase activity. Overexpression of S18-2 induced chromosomal instability in REF and also in the terminally differentiated rat skin fibroblast (Darekar et al., 2015).

RB forms a complex with amphipathic helix protein SIN3A (SIN3 transcription regulator family member A), along with SKI and HDAC (Tokitou et al., 1999). SIN3A controls the homeostasis by regulating the expression of MYC. SIN3A binds to MYC and causes deacetylation of MYC, which targets the latter for degradation (Nascimento et al., 2011). In the absence of SIN3A, MYC is recruited to epidermal differentiation complex, and reactivation of MYC target genes drives abnormal epidermal differentiation and proliferation. However, simultaneous inactivation of both *MYC* and *SIN3A* revert the aberrant skin phenotype to normal. SIN3A also antagonizes MYC oncogenic activities by interacting with MXI1 (Max-interacting protein 1) to repress MYC responsive genes (Rao et al., 1996). SIN3A is also an inhibitor of HDAC1 and HDAC2, and SIN3A-associated HDAC1 and HDAC2 are pivotal for the homeostasis of HSCs (Heideman et al., 2014).

TRAP1 (tumor necrosis factor receptor-associated protein 1) binds to hypophosphorylated RB, using LXCXE motif (Chen, Chen, et al., 1996). The overexpression of TRAP1 decreased apoptosis in NSCs and preserved mitochondrial membrane potential. Ectopic expression of TRAP1 resisted the neurotoxicity-mediated mitochondrial dysfunction by inhibiting the formation of cyclophilin D (CypD)-dependent mitochondrial permeability transition pore (mPTP). TRAP1 overexpression prevents the

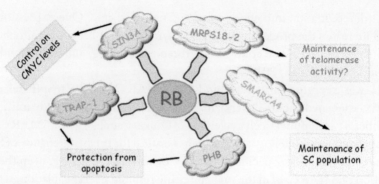

Fig. 6 RB is involved in control on tissue homeostasis. RB binds to proteins implicated in protection of apoptosis, maintenance of telomere length and SC population. *Blue* shapes (*wavy*) show binding between RB and discussed proteins. (See the color plate.)

impairment of NSCs induced by microglia–derived soluble factors that regulate the opening of mPTP (Wang et al., 2015) (Fig. 6).

9. CONCLUDING REMARKS

The capability of SCs to self-renew and to differentiate provides a vast potential for the treatment of cancer disease because they give rise to the different cell types and tissues in the body. Pluripotent SCs can be induced also from somatic cells, generating cells and tissues for transplantation. SCs might be of benefit for the drug research: drugs can be tested on cells generated from SCs, before using the animal models.

Despite of large number of studies devoted to SCs research, still the basic knowledge/understanding about the molecular mechanisms of SC biology is lacking. RB is an important protein for the normal physiology and survival of all kind of cells in the body. The present work encompasses 27 binding partners of RB protein that are involved in different physiological processes of SCs, including cell division, stemness, differentiation, and homeostasis. This study might be useful to further investigate and understand the behavior of SCs and their efficacy in the clinical use.

ACKNOWLEDGMENTS

Our work was supported by the Swedish Cancer Society, by matching grants from the Concern Foundation (Los Angeles) and the Cancer Research Institute (New York), and by the Swedish Institute. The funders had no role in the study design, data collection and analysis, decision to publish or preparation of this chapter.

Conflict of interests: None declared.

REFERENCES

Ashe, M., Pabon-Pena, L., Dees, E., Price, K. L., & Bader, D. (2004). LEK1 is a potential inhibitor of pocket protein-mediated cellular processes. *The Journal of Biological Chemistry*, *279*, 664–676.

Balasenthil, S., & Vadlamudi, R. K. (2003). Functional interactions between the estrogen receptor coactivator PELP1/MNAR and retinoblastoma protein. *The Journal of Biological Chemistry*, *278*, 22119–22127.

Becker, K. A., Ghule, P. N., Therrien, J. A., Lian, J. B., Stein, J. L., van Wijnen, A. J., et al. (2006). Self-renewal of human embryonic stem cells is supported by a shortened G1 cell cycle phase. *Journal of Cellular Physiology*, *209*, 883–893.

Benevolenskaya, E. V., Murray, H. L., Branton, P., Young, R. A., & Kaelin, W. G., Jr. (2005). Binding of pRB to the PHD protein RBP2 promotes cellular differentiation. *Molecular Cell*, *18*, 623–635.

Bergh, G., Ehinger, M., Olsson, I., Jacobsen, S. E., & Gullberg, U. (1999). Involvement of the retinoblastoma protein in monocytic and neutrophilic lineage commitment of human bone marrow progenitor cells. *Blood*, *94*, 1971–1978.

Blank, U., Karlsson, G., Moody, J. L., Utsugisawa, T., Magnusson, M., Singbrant, S., et al. (2006). Smad7 promotes self-renewal of hematopoietic stem cells. *Blood*, *108*, 4246–4254.

Brehm, A., Miska, E. A., McCance, D. J., Reid, J. L., Bannister, A. J., & Kouzarides, T. (1998). Retinoblastoma protein recruits histone deacetylase to repress transcription. *Nature*, *391*, 597–601.

Chen, C. F., Chen, Y., Dai, K., Chen, P. L., Riley, D. J., & Lee, W. H. (1996). A new member of the hsp90 family of molecular chaperones interacts with the retinoblastoma protein during mitosis and after heat shock. *Molecular and Cellular Biology*, *16*, 4691–4699.

Chen, P. L., Riley, D. J., Chen-Kiang, S., & Lee, W. H. (1996). Retinoblastoma protein directly interacts with and activates the transcription factor NF-IL6. *Proceedings of the National Academy of Sciences of the United States of America*, *93*, 465–469.

Classon, M., Kennedy, B. K., Mulloy, R., & Harlow, E. (2000). Opposing roles of pRB and p107 in adipocyte differentiation. *Proceedings of the National Academy of Sciences of the United States of America*, *97*, 10826–10831.

Conklin, J. F., Baker, J., & Sage, J. (2012). The RB family is required for the self-renewal and survival of human embryonic stem cells. *Nature Communications*, *3*, 1244–1255.

Corsini, N. S., Sancho-Martinez, I., Laudenklos, S., Glagow, D., Kumar, S., Letellier, E., et al. (2009). The death receptor CD95 activates adult neural stem cells for working memory formation and brain repair. *Cell Stem Cell*, *5*, 178–190.

Darekar, S. D., Mushtaq, M., Gurrapu, S., Kovalevska, L., Drummond, C., Petruchek, M., et al. (2015). Mitochondrial ribosomal protein S18-2 evokes chromosomal instability and transforms primary rat skin fibroblasts. *Oncotarget*, *6*, 21016–21028.

Deheuninck, J., & Luo, K. (2009). Ski and SnoN, potent negative regulators of TGF-beta signaling. *Cell Research*, *19*, 47–57.

Dunaief, J. L., Strober, B. E., Guha, S., Khavari, P. A., Alin, K., Luban, J., et al. (1994). The retinoblastoma protein and BRG1 form a complex and cooperate to induce cell cycle arrest. *Cell*, *79*, 119–310.

Endoh, M., Endo, T. A., Endoh, T., Fujimura, Y., Ohara, O., Toyoda, T., et al. (2008). Polycomb group proteins Ring1A/B are functionally linked to the core transcriptional regulatory circuitry to maintain ES cell identity. *Development*, *135*, 1513–1524.

Esterlechner, J., Reichert, N., Iltzsche, F., Krause, M., Finkernagel, F., & Gaubatz, S. (2013). LIN9, a subunit of the DREAM complex, regulates mitotic gene expression and proliferation of embryonic stem cells. *PloS One*, *8*, e62882.

Fang, F., Xu, Y., Chew, K. K., Chen, X., Ng, H. H., & Matsudaira, P. (2014). Coactivators p300 and CBP maintain the identity of mouse embryonic stem cells by mediating long-range chromatin structure. *Stem Cells*, *32*, 1805–1816.

Ferron, S. R., Pozo, N., Laguna, A., Aranda, S., Porlan, E., Moreno, M., et al. (2010). Regulated segregation of kinase Dyrk1A during asymmetric neural stem cell division is critical for EGFR-mediated biased signaling. *Cell Stem Cell, 7*, 367–379.

Gagrica, S., Hauser, S., Kolfschoten, I., Osterloh, L., Agami, R., & Gaubatz, S. (2004). Inhibition of oncogenic transformation by mammalian Lin-9, a pRB-associated protein. *The EMBO Journal, 23*, 4627–4638.

Galderisi, U., Cipollaro, M., & Giordano, A. (2006). The retinoblastoma gene is involved in multiple aspects of stem cell biology. *Oncogene, 25*, 5250–5256.

Gering, M., Yamada, Y., Rabbitts, T. H., & Patient, R. K. (2003). Lmo2 and Scl/Tal1 convert non-axial mesoderm into haemangioblasts which differentiate into endothelial cells in the absence of Gata1. *Development, 130*, 6187–6199.

Giacinti, C., & Giordano, A. (2006). RB and cell cycle progression. *Oncogene, 25*, 5220–5227.

Goodrich, D. W. (2006). The retinoblastoma tumor-suppressor gene, the exception that proves the rule. *Oncogene, 25*, 5233–5243.

Gu, W., Schneider, J. W., Condorelli, G., Kaushal, S., Mahdavi, V., & Nadal-Ginard, B. (1993). Interaction of myogenic factors and the retinoblastoma protein mediates muscle cell commitment and differentiation. *Cell, 72*, 309–324.

Heideman, M. R., Lancini, C., Proost, N., Yanover, E., Jacobs, H., & Dannenberg, J. H. (2014). Sin3a-associated Hdac1 and Hdac2 are essential for hematopoietic stem cell homeostasis and contribute differentially to hematopoiesis. *Haematologica, 99*, 1292–1303.

Hirama, T., & Koeffler, H. P. (1995). Role of the cyclin-dependent kinase inhibitors in the development of cancer. *Blood, 86*, 841–854.

Holik, A. Z., Krzystyniak, J., Young, M., Richardson, K., Jarde, T., Chambon, P., et al. (2013). Brg1 is required for stem cell maintenance in the murine intestinal epithelium in a tissue-specific manner. *Stem Cells, 31*, 2457–24669.

Hunter, T., & Pines, J. (1994). Cyclins and cancer. II: Cyclin D and CDK inhibitors come of age. *Cell, 79*, 573–582.

Jeon, B. N., Yoo, J. Y., Choi, W. I., Lee, C. E., Yoon, H. G., & Hur, M. W. (2008). Proto-oncogene FBI-1 (Pokemon/ZBTB7A) represses transcription of the tumor suppressor Rb gene via binding competition with Sp1 and recruitment of co-repressors. *The Journal of Biological Chemistry, 283*, 33199–33210.

Kashuba, E., Pavan Yenamandra, S., Darekar, S. D., Yurchenko, M., Kashuba, V., Klein, G., et al. (2009). MRPS18-2 protein immortalizes primary rat embryonic fibroblasts and endows them with stem cell-like properties. *Proceedings of the National Academy of Sciences of the United States of America, 106*, 19866–19871.

Kashuba, E., Yurchenko, M., Yenamandra, S. P., Snopok, B., Isaguliants, M., Szekely, L., et al. (2008). EBV-encoded EBNA-6 binds and targets MRS18-2 to the nucleus, resulting in the disruption of pRb-E2F1 complexes. *Proceedings of the National Academy of Sciences of the United States of America, 105*, 5489–5494.

Kim, Y. W., Otterson, G. A., Kratzke, R. A., Coxon, A. B., & Kaye, F. J. (1994). Differential specificity for binding of retinoblastoma binding protein 2 to RB, p107, and TATA-binding protein. *Molecular and Cellular Biology, 14*, 7256–7264.

Klose, R. J., Yan, Q., Tothova, Z., Yamane, K., Erdjument-Bromage, H., Tempst, P., et al. (2007). The retinoblastoma binding protein RBP2 is an H3K4 demethylase. *Cell, 128*, 889–900.

Kowno, M., Watanabe-Susaki, K., Ishimine, H., Komazaki, S., Enomoto, K., Seki, Y., et al. (2014). Prohibitin 2 regulates the proliferation and lineage-specific differentiation of mouse embryonic stem cells in mitochondria. *PloS One, 9*, e81552.

Kretsovali, A., Hadjimichael, C., & Charmpilas, N. (2012). Histone deacetylase inhibitors in cell pluripotency, differentiation, and reprogramming. *Stem Cells International, 184154*, 8–17.

Lavender, P., Vandel, L., Bannister, A. J., & Kouzarides, T. (1997). The HMG-box transcription factor HBP1 is targeted by the pocket proteins and E1A. *Oncogene, 14*, 2721–2728.

Lee, S. U., Maeda, M., Ishikawa, Y., Li, S. M., Wilson, A., Jubb, A. M., et al. (2013). LRF-mediated Dll4 repression in erythroblasts is necessary for hematopoietic stem cell maintenance. *Blood, 121*, 918–929.

Li, L. Q., Jothi, R., Cui, K., Lee, J. Y., Cohen, T., Gorivodsky, M., et al. (2011). Nuclear adaptor Ldb1 regulates a transcriptional program essential for the maintenance of hematopoietic stem cells. *Nature Immunology, 12*, 129–136.

Li, J., & Tsai, M. D. (2002). Novel insights into the INK4-CDK4/6-Rb pathway: Counter action of gankyrin against INK4 proteins regulates the CDK4-mediated phosphorylation of Rb. *Biochemistry, 41*, 3977–3983.

MacLellan, W. R., Xiao, G., Abdellatif, M., & Schneider, M. D. (2000). A novel Rb- and p300-binding protein inhibits transactivation by MyoD. *Molecular and Cellular Biology, 20*, 8903–8915.

Mead, P. E., Deconinck, A. E., Huber, T. L., Orkin, S. H., & Zon, L. I. (2001). Primitive erythropoiesis in the Xenopus embryo: The synergistic role of LMO-2, SCL and GATA-binding proteins. *Development, 128*, 2301–2308.

Mine, H., Sakurai, T., Kashida, H., Matsui, S., Nishida, N., Nagai, T., et al. (2013). Association of gankyrin and stemness factor expression in human colorectal cancer. *Digestive Diseases and Sciences, 58*, 2337–2344.

Mittnacht, S. (2005). The retinoblastoma protein—From bench to bedside. *European Journal of Cell Biology, 84*, 97–107.

Morgan, D. O. (1995). Principles of CDK regulation. *Nature, 374*, 131–134.

Mori, T., Ikeda, D. D., Fukushima, T., Takenoshita, S., & Kochi, H. (2011). NIRF constitutes a nodal point in the cell cycle network and is a candidate tumor suppressor. *Cell Cycle, 10*, 3284–3299.

Nam, C. H., & Rabbitts, T. H. (2006). The role of LMO2 in development and in T cell leukemia after chromosomal translocation or retroviral insertion. *Molecular Therapy, 13*, 15–25.

Nascimento, E. M., Cox, C. L., MacArthur, S., Hussain, S., Trotter, M., Blanco, S., et al. (2011). The opposing transcriptional functions of Sin3A and c-Myc are required to maintain tissue homeostasis. *Nature Cell Biology, 13*, 1395–1405.

Nicol, R., & Stavnezer, E. (1998). Transcriptional repression by v-Ski and c-Ski mediated by a specific DNA binding site. *The Journal of Biological Chemistry, 273*, 3588–3597.

Novitch, B. G., Mulligan, G. J., Jacks, T., & Lassar, A. B. (1996). Skeletal muscle cells lacking the retinoblastoma protein display defects in muscle gene expression and accumulate in S and G2 phases of the cell cycle. *The Journal of Cell Biology, 135*, 441–456.

Pichler, G., Wolf, P., Schmidt, C. S., Meilinger, D., Schneider, K., Frauer, C., et al. (2011). Cooperative DNA and histone binding by Uhrf2 links the two major repressive epigenetic pathways. *Journal of Cellular Biochemistry, 112*, 2585–2593.

Pradhan, S., & Kim, G. D. (2002). The retinoblastoma gene product interacts with maintenance human DNA (cytosine-5) methyltransferase and modulates its activity. *The EMBO Journal, 21*, 779–788.

Rao, G., Alland, L., Guida, P., Schreiber-Agus, N., Chen, K., Chin, L., et al. (1996). Mouse Sin3A interacts with and can functionally substitute for the amino-terminal repression of the Myc antagonist Mxi1. *Oncogene, 12*, 1165–1172.

Ryall, J. G., Dell'Orso, S., Derfoul, A., Juan, A., Zare, H., Feng, X., et al. (2015). The NAD(+)-dependent SIRT1 deacetylase translates a metabolic switch into regulatory epigenetics in skeletal muscle stem cells. *Cell Stem Cell, 16*, 171–183.

Sage, J. (2012). The retinoblastoma tumor suppressor and stem cell biology. *Genes & Development, 26*, 1409–1420.

Schwaller, J., Pabst, T., Koeffler, H. P., Niklaus, G., Loetscher, P., Fey, M. F., et al. (1997). Expression and regulation of G1 cell-cycle inhibitors (p16INK4A, p15INK4B, p18INK4C, p19INK4D) in human acute myeloid leukemia and normal myeloid cells. *Leukemia, 11*, 54–63.

Sherr, C. J. (1993). Mammalian G1 cyclins. *Cell, 73*, 1059–1065.

Singbrant, S., Wall, M., Moody, J., Karlsson, G., Chalk, A. M., Liddicoat, B., et al. (2014). The SKI proto-oncogene enhances the in vivo repopulation of hematopoietic stem cells and causes myeloproliferative disease. *Haematologica, 99*, 647–655.

Toguchida, J., McGee, T. L., Paterson, J. C., Eagle, J. R., Tucker, S., Yandell, D. W., et al. (1993). Complete genomic sequence of the human retinoblastoma susceptibility gene. *Genomics, 17*, 535–543.

Tokitou, F., Nomura, T., Khan, M. M., Kaul, S. C., Wadhwa, R., Yasukawa, T., et al. (1999). Viral ski inhibits retinoblastoma protein (Rb)-mediated transcriptional repression in a dominant negative fashion. *The Journal of Biological Chemistry, 274*, 4485–4488.

Trowbridge, J. J., Snow, J. W., Kim, J., & Orkin, S. H. (2009). DNA methyltransferase 1 is essential for and uniquely regulates hematopoietic stem and progenitor cells. *Cell Stem Cell, 5*, 442–449.

van der Stoop, P., Boutsma, E. A., Hulsman, D., Noback, S., Heimerikx, M., Kerkhoven, R. M., et al. (2008). Ubiquitin E3 ligase Ring1b/Rnf2 of polycomb repressive complex 1 contributes to stable maintenance of mouse embryonic stem cells. *PloS One, 3*, e0002235.

Varjosalo, M., Keskitalo, S., Van Drogen, A., Nurkkala, H., Vichalkovski, A., Aebersold, R., et al. (2013). The protein interaction landscape of the human CMGC kinase group. *Cell Reports, 3*, 1306–1320.

Vitelli, L., Condorelli, G., Lulli, V., Hoang, T., Luchetti, L., Croce, C. M., et al. (2000). A pentamer transcriptional complex including tal-1 and retinoblastoma protein downmodulates c-kit expression in normal erythroblasts. *Molecular and Cellular Biology, 20*, 5330–5342.

Voncken, J. W., Roelen, B. A., Roefs, M., de Vries, S., Verhoeven, E., Marino, S., et al. (2003). Rnf2 (Ring1b) deficiency causes gastrulation arrest and cell cycle inhibition. *Proceedings of the National Academy of Sciences of the United States of America, 100*, 2468–2473.

Wang, C., Chen, L., Hou, X., Li, Z., Kabra, N., Ma, Y., et al. (2006). Interactions between E2F1 and SirT1 regulate apoptotic response to DNA damage. *Nature Cell Biology, 8*, 1025–1031.

Wang, Y., Lin, J., Chen, Q. Z., Zhu, N., Jiang, D. Q., & Li, M. X. (2015). Overexpression of mitochondrial Hsp75 protects neural stem cells against microglia-derived soluble factor-induced neurotoxicity by regulating mitochondrial permeability transition pore opening in vitro. *International Journal of Molecular Medicine, 36*, 1487–1496.

Wang, S., Nath, N., Adlam, M., & Chellappan, S. (1999). Prohibitin, a potential tumor suppressor, interacts with RB and regulates E2F function. *Oncogene, 18*, 3501–3510.

Wang, J., Qiang, Z., Song, S., Shi, L., Ma, C., & Tan, X. (2013). Temporal expression of Pelp1 during proliferation and osteogenic differentiation of rat bone marrow mesenchymal stem cells. *PloS One, 8*, e75477.

Warren, A. J., Colledge, W. H., Carlton, M. B., Evans, M. J., Smith, A. J., & Rabbitts, T. H. (1994). The oncogenic cysteine-rich LIM domain protein rbtn2 is essential for erythroid development. *Cell, 78*, 45–57.

Watanabe, N., Kageyama, R., & Ohtsuka, T. (2015). Hbp1 regulates the timing of neuronal differentiation during cortical development by controlling cell cycle progression. *Development, 142*, 2278–2290.

Weinberg, R. A. (2007). The biology of cancer. In E. Jeffcock (Ed.), *Vol. 1* (pp. 255–300). USA: Garland Science, Taylor and Francis Group.

Welinder, E., & Murre, C. (2011). Ldb1, a new guardian of hematopoietic stem cell maintenance. *Nature Immunology, 12*, 113–114.

Yan, X. Q., Sarmiento, U., Sun, Y., Huang, G., Guo, J., Juan, T., et al. (2001). A novel Notch ligand, Dll4, induces T-cell leukemia/lymphoma when overexpressed in mice by retroviral-mediated gene transfer. *Blood, 98*, 3793–3799.

Yenamandra, S. P., Darekar, S. D., Kashuba, V., Matskova, L., Klein, G., & Kashuba, E. (2012). Stem cell gene expression in MRPS18-2-immortalized rat embryonic fibroblasts. *Cell Death & Disease, 19*, 138.

Yi, F., Pereira, L., Hoffman, J. A., Shy, B. R., Yuen, C. M., Liu, D. R., et al. (2011). Opposing effects of Tcf3 and Tcf1 control Wnt stimulation of embryonic stem cell self-renewal. *Nature Cell Biology, 13*, 762–770.

Zhu, L. (2005). Tumour suppressor retinoblastoma protein Rb: A transcriptional regulator. *European Journal of Cancer, 41*, 2415–2427.

CHAPTER SIX

Evolving Strategies for Therapeutically Targeting Cancer Stem Cells

S. Talukdar*, L. Emdad*,†,‡, S.K. Das*,†,‡, D. Sarkar*,†,‡, P.B. Fisher*,†,‡,1

*Virginia Commonwealth University, School of Medicine, Richmond, VA, United States
†VCU Institute of Molecular Medicine, Virginia Commonwealth University, School of Medicine, Richmond, VA, United States
‡VCU Massey Cancer Center, Virginia Commonwealth University, School of Medicine, Richmond, VA, United States
1Corresponding author: e-mail address: paul.fisher@vcuhealth.org

Contents

Abstract

Cancer is a multifactor and multistep process that is affected intrinsically by the genetic and epigenetic makeup of tumor cells and extrinsically by the host microenvironment and immune system. A key component of cancer involves a unique subpopulation of

Advances in Cancer Research, Volume 131
ISSN 0065-230X
http://dx.doi.org/10.1016/bs.acr.2016.04.003

highly malignant cancerous cells referred to as cancer stem cells (CSCs). CSCs are positioned at the apex of the tumor hierarchy with an ability to both self-renew and also generate non-CSC/differentiated progeny, which contribute to the majority of the tumor mass. CSCs undergo functional changes and show plasticity that is stimulated by specific microenvironmental cues and interactions in the tumor niche, which contribute to the complexity and heterogeneity of the CSC population. The prognostic value of CSCs in the clinic is evident since there are many examples in which CSCs serve as markers for poor patient prognosis. CSCs are innately resistant to many standard therapies and they display anoikis resistance, immune evasion, tumor dormancy, and field cancerization, which may result in metastasis and relapse. Many academic laboratories and biotechnology companies are currently focusing on strategies that target CSCs. Combination therapies, epigenetic modifiers, stemness inhibitors, CSC surface marker-based therapies, and immunotherapy-based CSC-targeting drugs are currently undergoing clinical trials. Potential new targets/strategies in CSC-targeted therapy include MDA-9/Syntenin (SDCBP), Patched (PTCH), epigenetic targets, noncoding RNAs, and differentiation induction. Defining ways of targeting and destroying CSCs holds potential to impact significantly on cancer therapy, including prevention of metastasis and cancer recurrence.

1. INTRODUCTION

1.1 Cancer Stem Cell Concept

The existence of cancer stem cells (CSCs) is a relatively recent concept, which suggests that tumor growth is sustained by a subpopulation of highly malignant cancerous cells (Baccelli & Trumpp, 2012). These cells are at the top of the tumor pyramid, possessing self-renewing potential, quiescent or slow–cycling states, and increased resistance to conventional therapies. Currently, most studies indicate that the cellular and molecular events leading to tumor initiation are orchestrated by CSC–like cells (Bjerkvig, Tysnes, Aboody, Najbauer, & Terzis, 2005). The involvement of CSCs in the generation of cancer is a component of every major theory of the origin of cancer including field theory, chemical carcinogenesis, infection, mutation, or epigenetic changes (Sell, 2010). CSCs may originate from self-renewing stem cells or from more differentiated progenitors that develop stemness traits by accrual of genetic and/or epigenetic aberrations (Baccelli & Trumpp, 2012). The tumor cell of origin delineates the specific cell type involved, which could be the initial cell type first affected by an oncogenic mutation. However, this cell of origin may not automatically acquire a CSC phenotype (Visvader & Lindeman, 2012). It is entirely possible for a tumor to have multiple cells of origin and be comprised of multiple different CSC types (Fig. 1). Although the genetic and CSC models of cancer are often studied as mutually exclusive models for tumor heterogeneity, it has been proposed that both can be standardized by considering the role of genetic diversity and nongenetic influences in contributing to tumor heterogeneity (Kreso & Dick, 2014).

1.2 Tumor Hierarchy, Heterogeneity, and Plasticity

The master regulatory transcription factors and their downstream mediators, discussed later in this review, are recognized drivers of the hierarchical organization of stem and progenitor cells and their differentiated progeny during development. Some cancer types also depend on analogous cellular hierarchies. CSCs are capable of generating the full spectrum of cell types present in a tumor. Positioned at the zenith of the tumor pyramid, CSCs can not only self-renew but also generate non–CSC/differentiated progeny, which comprises the main body of the tumor (Baccelli & Trumpp, 2012). This hierarchical tumor organization, directed by CSCs, has been reported for several tumor types such as germ cell cancers, leukemia, breast cancer, brain cancer, colon cancer, pancreatic cancer, melanoma, and several other tumor indications (Baccelli & Trumpp, 2012). Additional mutations can change the properties of CSCs as well as differentiated progeny, and new CSCs can also appear in the tumor, adding to complexity (Baccelli & Trumpp, 2012; Fig. 1). CSC plasticity adds yet another level of complexity. This fluid process underlies the dynamic ability of cancer cells to shift from a non–CSC state to a CSC state and vice versa, which may be modulated by specific microenvironmental signals and cellular interactions developing in the tumor niche (Cabrera, Hollingsworth, & Hurt, 2015). This process suggests a revision to the earlier CSC concept that only the tumorigenic subset in the tumor needs to be targeted. Through an appreciation of the interrelationship between CSCs and their differentiated progeny, it may be possible to design better therapeutic regimens that can prevent the development of metastases and relapse (Tang, 2012).

1.3 Microenvironment and Niche Interactions with CSCs

The tumor niche or microenvironment is an intricate network of cells, signaling molecules, soluble factors, and the extracellular matrix that plays an essential role in tumor development, metastasis, and therapeutic response (Cabrera et al., 2015). The microenvironmental factors include signaling molecules, hematopoietic cells, stromal cells, inflammatory cells,

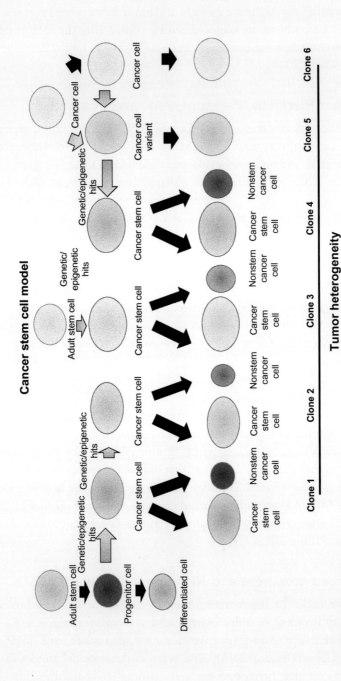

Fig. 1 Schematic representation of the cancer stem cell concept. (See the color plate.)

vasculature, and the extracellular matrix (Cabrera et al., 2015). Each of these cellular and noncellular factors contributes not only to the transformation of tumor cells but also regulates response to chemotherapy and radiation treatments by providing protection from these agents (Cabrera et al., 2015). CSC function and plasticity may also be stimulated by specific microenvironmental cues and interactions in the tumor niche (Cabrera et al., 2015). NOTCH, Hedgehog, and hypoxia-inducible factor are some of the signaling molecules implicated as niche-derived signals that maintain the CSC phenotype (Cabrera et al., 2015). Disrupting CSCs and/or their molecular crosstalk with other niche constituents is very critical for effectively blocking tumor progression (Squadrito & De Palma, 2015). Vascular niche has also been implicated in maintaining tumor dormancy, providing another level of complexity (Ghajar, 2015).

1.4 Clinical Significance of CSCs

1.4.1 Prognostic Outcome

CSCs have been isolated from leukemia, breast, prostate, brain, pancreatic, colon, and other types of cancer using either cell surface marker-based (eg, CD44+, CD24−, CD133+, etc.) or dye-efflux-based side population identification combined with cell sorting (Tu, Foltz, Lin, Hood, & Tian, 2009). The prognostic value of CSC markers in the clinic is expanding, since it has been shown that CSCs are markers for poor patient prognosis (Ailles & Weissman, 2007; Kawasaki & Farrar, 2008). It is now established that certain brain CSCs are particularly resistant to radiotherapy (Bao et al., 2006; Kawasaki & Farrar, 2008). CSCs are now deemed responsible for acute myeloid leukemia (AML) persistence and recurrence following cytotoxic or targeted therapy; and presence of additional markers such as CD33, $t(8;21)$, $t(15;17)$, and monosomy seven can predict response to chemotherapy in AML (Tu et al., 2009). Comparison of a 186-gene expression profile of CD44+/CD24−/low putative breast CSCs to that of normal breast epithelium revealed a significant association between this gene signature in both overall and metastasis-free survival ($P < 0.001$) that was unbiased by established clinical and pathological variables (Tu et al., 2009). The unique gene signature further stratified patients into high-risk (10-year survival of 81%) and low-risk (10-year survival of 57%, $P = 0.01$) groups. These gene signatures are also linked with the prognosis in medulloblastoma ($P = 0.004$), lung cancer ($P = 0.03$), and prostate cancer ($P = 0.01$) (Liu et al., 2007; Tu et al., 2009).

The prognostic value of CD133 has also been the focus of many studies. High CD133 expression correlated with poor clinical outcomes in glioma, colon cancer, prostate, and head neck cancer (Tu et al., 2009). Increased CD133, CD90, CD44, CD24, EpCAM, and Nestin expression and lack of CD45 expression have also proven to be prognostic factors for survival and tumor recurrence in patients with hepatocellular carcinoma (Ji & Wang, 2012; Tu et al., 2009). CSC generation capability and presence of even 2% CD133+ cells in glioblastoma (GBM) lesions negatively correlated with overall ($P=0.0001$ and 0.02, respectively) and progression-free ($P=0.0002$ and 0.01, respectively) survival of patients (Balbous et al., 2014; Pallini et al., 2008). Balbous et al. performed expression profiling analysis of pluripotency in gliomaspheres derived from 11 patients. A stable pattern for SOX2 was observed suggesting its potential relevance in maintaining pluripotency in GSCs. All GSC samples used in this study were shown to have the capacity to commit to neural differentiation and express mesenchymal or endothelial differentiation markers (Balbous et al., 2014). They also found that expression of COL1A1 and IFITM1 genes could stratify patients with GBM into subgroups for risk of recurrence at diagnosis, as well as for prognostic and therapeutic response (Balbous et al., 2014).

CSCs in inflammatory breast cancer were found to be an independent predictive variable for early metastasis development and decreased survival (Charafe-Jauffret et al., 2010). Studies on CSC markers for colorectal cancer have been controversial; stem cells taken from patients with tumors harboring higher levels of both CD44 and CD133 had a higher risk of developing early liver metastases, whereas other studies showed that knock-down of CD44 expression resulted in almost a 10-fold increase in metastatic potential in both the liver and the lungs and low levels of CD44 were relevant for increased tumor relapse and short disease-free survival in colon cancer patients (Kim, 2015). Other studies have concluded that colon cancer patients expressing high ALCAM levels display poor clinical outcome (Kim, 2015). The conflicting data could be a consequence of genetic and epigenetic effects on the expression of CSC surface markers. Validation of different markers for each cancer type in independent cohorts as a diagnostic prediction model is essential before these markers can be utilized clinically.

1.4.2 Chemoresistance

An ominous outcome of the presence of CSCs is that these cells may be innately resistant to many standard modes of therapy (Dean, 2009).

Accumulating evidence supports the concept that CSCs are intrinsically resistant to chemotherapy via their relative quiescence, enhanced DNA repair ability, ABC transporter expression, and reduced entry into apoptosis. Using these mechanisms some CSCs survive therapy and bring about relapse, even many years after therapy (Dean, 2009). Clonal evolution of CSCs may also give rise to tumors in which all the cells display a multidrug resistance (MDR) phenotype, a major cause of relapse. MDR is a major barrier to effective cancer therapy and is considered to be a major contributor to cancer-related death along with metastasis. Elucidation of the molecular basis of MDR and developing clinical reagents or strategies to prevent and treat MDR tumors is a high priority. The P-glycoprotein encoded by the ABCB1 gene was the first and the best characterized ABC transporter identified to be amplified and/or overexpressed in MDR tumor cell lines (Dean, 2009; Roninson et al., 1986). There are a wide variety of clinical agents that inhibit ABCB1 that have been evaluated in clinical studies against cancer, however, none of these clinical trials were very positive (Crowley, McDevitt, & Callaghan, 2010; Dean, 2009; Tarasova et al., 2005). Nevertheless, there are several ABC proteins widely overexpressed in tumor cells, such as ABCC1/MRP1 and ABCG2. The finding that there are multiple potential efflux pumps that a cell can employ for MDR, increases the complexity of appropriate targeting. The ABC transporters also play significant roles in drug distribution as they provide important functions in compound access across the blood–brain barrier, intestine, and other tissues compartments (Dean, 2009; Doyle et al., 1998). Gaining a better insight into the mechanisms of stem cell resistance to chemotherapy has potential to lead to new therapeutic targets and improved anticancer strategies (Dean, 2009).

1.4.3 Radiation Resistance

There is growing evidence that CSCs are innately resistant to radiation, by regulating the repair of DNA damage, redistribution of cells in the cell cycle, increased activation of the DNA damage checkpoint, repopulation, and reoxygenation of hypoxic tumor areas (Pajonk, Vlashi, & McBride, 2010; Rich, 2007). Recent studies showed that induced breast cancer stem cells (iBCSCs) were produced by radiation-induced activation of the same cellular pathways utilized to reprogram normal cells into induced pluripotent stem cells in regenerative medicine (Lagadec, Vlashi, Della Donna, Dekmezian, & Pajonk, 2012). Significant correlations have been found between radiation therapy clinical outcomes and circulating CSCs (Kurth et al., 2015; McInnes et al., 2015). Confusing factors remaining constant, the radiation dose to eradicate a tumor inversely correlates with the log number of CSCs (Krause, Dubrovska, Linge, & Baumann, 2016). Significantly high DNA repair abilities have been observed in CSC populations from different cancers such as glioblastoma, prostate, lung, and breast cancers and this is mostly attributed to the activation of the ATR-Chk1 and ATM-Chk2 signaling pathways (Krause et al., 2016). Radiotherapy leads to upregulation of prostate CSC markers and differentially regulates several relevant molecules/pathways including aldehyde dehydrogenase (ALDH) activity, OCT4, NANOG, BMI1, ATP-binding cassette subfamily G member 2 (ABCG2), phosphatidylinositide 3-kinases PI3K/AKT activation, and increased β-catenin and vimentin expression (Cojoc et al., 2015; Krause et al., 2016). A phenotypic switch during radiotherapy is activated by the presence of active histone methylation at the promoter sequence of the ALDH1A1 gene leading to higher tumorigenicity and radioresistance of the prostate cancer cells that underwent multiple irradiations (Cojoc et al., 2015). Similar observations have been reported for ALDH1A3 expression in head and neck cancer (Krause et al., 2016). Apart from a higher radioresistance of CSCs compared to non–CSC tumor cells, these outcomes can also be explained by production of new CSCs from previously nontumorigenic cells after irradiation (Lagadec et al., 2012; Pajonk & Vlashi, 2013). These effects are possibly a result of proinflammatory signaling within normal tissue cells of the tumor microenvironment after irradiation and/or hypoxic microenvironmental conditions (Krause et al., 2016; Mathieu et al., 2011; Schwitalla et al., 2013).

1.4.4 Dissemination/Anoikis Resistance

Metastasis is a complex process involving dissociation of cancer cells from their primary sites, survival in the vascular system, and subsequent attachment, invasion, and proliferation in distant target organs (Obenauf & Massagué, 2015; Oskarsson & Massagué, 2012). Normal cells undergo an apoptotic process called anoikis, after the loss of contact with the extracellular matrix or neighboring cells (Fofaria & Srivastava, 2015; Schempp et al., 2014; Simpson, Anyiwe, & Schimmer, 2008). Anoikis resistance is essential for cancer cells to endure the process of dissemination via the circulatory and lymphatic systems, after detachment from primary sites (Kim, Koo, Sung, Yun, & Kim, 2012). There is increasing evidence of a correlation between these anoikis-resistant circulating tumor cells and CSCs (Kantara et al., 2015; Katoh et al., 2015; Scatena, Bottoni, & Giardina, 2013; Toloudi, Apostolou,

Chatziioannou, & Papasotiriou, 2011). Detection of anoikis-resistant circulating tumor cells is currently an active area of cancer research. Studies focusing on CSC-targeting potential of apoptosis-targeted therapies and
mechanisms of apoptosis-resistance in these cells are limited (Kruyt &
Schuringa, 2010). Detailed molecular and functional studies of anoikis-
resistant CSCs may provide an enhanced understanding of the biology of
cancer metastasis as well as help identify novel therapeutic targets for prevention of cancer dissemination (Kim et al., 2012). Anoikis resistance may be
regulated by both intrinsic and extrinsic factors including the differentiation
status of stem cells, exogenous environmental factors, microenvironmental
survival factors, and hypoxic conditions (Kruyt & Schuringa, 2010). The initiation of an embryonic genetic program resulting in the transition from an
epithelial to a mesenchymal state (EMT) may also be responsible for anoikis
resistance in CSCs (Kruyt & Schuringa, 2010). Considering the plasticity
and niche interactions of CSCs, it is not known if a specific or single
apoptosis-inducing strategy could efficiently eliminate all CSCs (Frisch,
Schaller, & Cieply, 2013; Kruyt & Schuringa, 2010).

1.4.5 Immune Evasion

Evasion of the immune system is a prerequisite for tumor spread, progression, and recurrence. CSCs play a very important role in immune evasion
(Bruttel & Wischhusen, 2014; Kawasaki & Farrar, 2008). Immune evasion
or tumor tolerance is the ability of a tumor to escape recognition by the
immune system, thereby allowing transformed cells to grow, spread, and
proliferate at secondary sites (Kawasaki & Farrar, 2008; Wang & Fisher,
2015; Zou, 2005). CSCs may use this mechanism to escape detection by
the immune system. Recent studies indicate a negative correlation between
degrees of host immunocompetence and rates of cancer development, indicating that CSCs possess the phenotypic and functional characteristics
required to evade host antitumor immunity (Nahas, Patel, Bliss, &
Rameshwar, 2012; Schatton & Frank, 2009). Numerous immunosuppressive molecules have been identified including programmed cell death 1
(PD-1), programmed cell death 1 ligand 1 (PD1-L1), transforming growth
factor β (TGF-β), cytotoxic T-lymphocyte-associated 4 (CTLA-4), B- and
T-lymphocyte attenuator (BTLA) (Santarpia et al., 2015), and CD200
(Kawasaki & Farrar, 2008; Wang & Fisher, 2015; Wang, Zuo, Sarkar, &
Fisher, 2011). Immune selection also enhances the growth and stem-like
properties of tumor cells (Noh et al., 2012).

1.4.6 Dormancy

Many cancer patients undergo metastatic relapse even several years after radical surgery or chemotherapy treatment. Dissemination of anoikis resistant, circulating CSCs, followed by dormancy potentially explains this prevalent clinical behavior (Giancotti, 2013; Kim et al., 2012; Patel & Chen, 2012). There are also conspicuous similarities between the concept of tumor dormancy and CSCs (Kleffel & Schatton, 2013). In fact, quiescence and immune escape are two of the currently emerging signature characteristics of at least some CSCs, emphasizing a significant overlap between dormant cancer populations and CSCs (Kleffel & Schatton, 2013). Several studies indicate that metastasis–initiating dormant cells are in fact CSCs that revert to a functional active state upon infiltrating a target organ (Giancotti, 2013). Entry of CSCs into dormancy and their subsequent reactivation are regulated by intrinsic factors and appropriate extrinsic signals. Dormant cells undergoing reactivation are supported by specialized extracellular matrix niches, which enable positive signals, such as Wnt and NOTCH, and diminish negative signals, such as BMP (Giancotti, 2013). The purpose of dormancy in CSCs is possibly to activate stress responses to protect them from the suppressive or hostile target organ microenvironment and allow CSCs to survive in foreign tissues for an extended period of time (Patel & Chen, 2012). Furthermore, apart from a role in maintaining residual disease after treatment, dormancy could also support early stages of tumor development and the generation of clinically undetectable micrometastatic foci (Kleffel & Schatton, 2013). Acquisition of an environment-independent, intrinsic dormant state is an expected early obstacle to tumor progression (Enderling, 2013). The mechanisms regulating tumor dormancy still remain poorly understood, and this results in significant problems in the clinical management of cancer (Allan, Vantyghem, Tuck, & Chambers, 2006). Improved understanding of CSC-mediated tumor dormancy has the potential to uncover new therapeutic avenues to eliminate metastatic tumors and significantly decrease cancer mortality (Ghajar, 2015; Patel & Chen, 2012).

1.4.7 Field Cancerization

Field cancerization is the presence of transformed cells adjacent to the primary tumor, and it is hypothesized to be a mediator of disease progression and relapse (Simple, Suresh, Das, & Kuriakose, 2015). This process involves multiple intricate molecular events leading to the transformation of a completely normal cell into a cancer cell. CSCs are capable of tumor initiation and migration, both of which are necessary for regulating field cancerization (Simple et al., 2015). Loss of heterozygosity, microsatellite alterations, chromosomal instability, mutations in the TP53 gene, and telomerase activity are the established molecular markers used to differentiate and characterize CSC-mediated field cancerization (Simple et al., 2015). Cells expressing cancer-activated fibroblast markers show an abundant deposition of Tenascin C and Periostin, two interacting matricellular proteins that form CSC niches, and these may also be involved in the field cancerization process (Oskarsson & Massagué, 2012; Vanharanta & Massagué, 2012). Field cancerization is observed in several cancers and is an important factor in risk assessment, early cancer detection, monitoring tumor progression, and in the definition of tumor margins (Dakubo, Jakupciak, Birch-Machin, & Parr, 2007).

1.5 Hurdles and Approaches in CSC Targeting

Current anticancer therapies not only fail to eliminate CSC clones but instead, support the enrichment of the CSC pool by selecting for resistant clones culminating in resistance and subsequent relapse in these patients. The identification of CSC-specific marker subsets and the targeted therapeutic destruction of CSCs remain challenging endeavors (Leon, MacDonagh, Finn, Cuffe, & Barr, 2016). The tumor environment creates a favorable niche that not only supports the survival and proliferation of CSCs but also protects CSCs from chemotherapy-induced apoptosis and helps CSCs enter quiescent states as well as adapt to therapy (Besançon, Valsesia-Wittmann, Puisieux, Caron de Fromentel, & Maguer-Satta, 2009). Strategies targeting CSCs are critically important for developing new and effective therapeutic approaches for cancer (Leon et al., 2016). The inherent resistant nature of CSCs to therapy is also a potential factor leading to therapeutic toxicity in patients. Increased high dosage of multiple drugs or radiation causes severe side effects in patients. Targeting of these drugs specifically to the CSCs might provide a better strategy to mitigate some of the toxicity. However, CSC-specificity has been difficult to achieve, first due to the heterogeneous nature of cancer and second due to the presence of normal cells with the same cell surface molecules as CSCs. Systemic delivery of CSC-targeting drugs remains problematic because of the complex heterogeneity of CSCs and the surface antigenic similarity between normal and CSCs. For specific sites, such as the brain, delivery is challenging due to the presence of the blood–brain barrier. In principle, localized targeted delivery may provide better therapeutic outcomes.

Some clinical trials are evaluating the applicability and efficacy of NOTCH or Hedgehog pathway inhibitors together with palliative radiotherapy. However, it is too early to determine if these combinatorial approaches will yield positive outcomes (Krause et al., 2016). In the context of radiotherapy, it is essential to focus on chemotherapeutic combinations that are as specific as possible to CSCs with no or only minimal effects on surrounding normal tissues to avoid increased radiogenic toxicities to normal tissues (Krause et al., 2016). Bioavailability of the drugs to the CSCs, which may be located in hypoxic niches with little or no blood perfusion is another area of concern. If the target of the drug is also expressed on non-CSCs close to a vessel along the diffusion path and/or if the plasma half-life of the drug is short, these could further exacerbate problems. These hurdles may lead to no discernible effects on CSCs in vivo, even if there are cytotoxic effects on CSCs in vitro (Krause et al., 2016).

2. CURRENT AND PIPELINE THERAPEUTIC TARGETS AND STRATEGIES

2.1 Chemotherapy and Radiotherapy

Chemotherapy and radiotherapy are currently the two "gold standards" of cancer treatment, and the resistance of CSCs to these treatments is well documented. Academicians and biotechnology companies are aggressively focusing on strategies that target CSCs. Verastem, a stem cell startup, procured $57 million in its initial public offering of stock, in spite of being a year away from clinical trials (http://www.businesswire.com/news/home/20150917005120/en/Verastem-Present-Preclinical-Data-ESMOECCO-2015; Schmidt, 2012). Japanese pharmaceutical giant Dainippon Sumitomo bought Boston Biomedical Inc. a biotech company with two anti-CSC agents in clinical trials, for $200 million down and almost $2.4 billion in milestone payments (Schmidt, 2012). Both events indicate escalating confidence in the importance of therapies directed against CSCs. There are several drugs currently in various stages of clinical trials, many of which are either inducers of CSC death, differentiation or target currently known stemness pathways (Table 1). Most of these drugs focus on targeting the NOTCH, Hedgehog, or Wnt signaling molecules (Takebe et al., 2015). However, the critical obstacle is to confirm that these drugs do not end up targeting the normal stem

Table 1 Drugs Targeting CSCs/CSC Pathways in Clinical Trials

Compound	Cancer Stem Cell	Mechanism	Clinical Trial	References
Salinomycin	Colon and breast	Apoptosis	Pilot clinical trial	Zhang et al. (2015)
Curcumin	Colon	Apoptosis and autophagy	Phase II	Zhang et al. (2015)
Torin-1	Colon	mTOR inhibition	Under trial	Zhang et al. (2015)
Rottlerin	Breast	do	Under trial	Zhang et al. (2015)
NVP-BEZ235	Glioma	do	Under trial	Zhang et al. (2015)
ITF2357	Lung	HDAC inhibition	Phase II	Zhang et al. (2015)
SAHA	Glioma	do	Phase II	Zhang et al. (2015)
Resveratrol	CSC	Apoptosis	Under trial	Zhang et al. (2015)
Metformin	Breast and pancreatic	Apoptosis	Phase III	Zhang et al. (2015)
Chloroquine	Breast Advanced solid tumors	Autophagy inhibition Combination with carboplatin and gemcitabine	Phase II Phase I	Lv and Shim (2015)
R737	Solid tumors	NRP1 targeting	Phase I	Schmidt (2012)
VS-5584	Solid tumors	PI3K/mTOR dual inhibitor	Escalation trial	Kolev et al. (2015)
SGT-53		CSC-targeting nanocomplex in combination with temozolomide	Under trial	Kim (2015)
VS-6063	Mesothelioma	FAK inhibition	Phase 1/1b	Pachter et al. (2015)

Continued

Table 1 Drugs Targeting CSCs/CSC Pathways in Clinical Trials—cont'd

Compound	Cancer Stem Cell	Mechanism	Clinical Trial	References
All-trans retinoic acid	Breast	CSC phenotype reversal to non-CSC	Preclinical	Bhat-Nakshatri, Goswami, Badve, Sledge, and Nakshatri (2013)
LF3	Colon	Wnt inhibition	Preclinical	Fang et al. (2016)
BBI608	Colorectal Ovarian, breast, nonsmall cell lung, melanoma, head and neck	Inhibits NANOG and other cancer stem cell pathways by targeting kinases	Phase III Phase Ib and II	Schmidt (2012)
BBI503	Solid tumor	Kinase inhibitor	Phase I	Schmidt (2012)
VS–507	Breast cancer	Wnt pathway	Under trial	Schmidt (2012)
VS-4718	Advanced breast cancer	FAK inhibitor	Phase 1	Schmidt (2012)
VS-5095	Breast cancer	FAK inhibitor	Preclinical	Schmidt (2012)
OMP-21M18/ Demcizumab	Solid tumor	NOTCH inhibitor	Phase Ib/II	Schmidt (2012)
BMS-986115	Solid tumor	NOTCH inhibitor	Under trial	Takebe et al. (2015)
MEDI0639	Solid tumor	Anti-DLL4 antibody	Under trial	Takebe et al. (2015)
OMP-59R5	Solid tumor, pancreatic cancer, SCLC	Anti-NOTCH2 antibody	Under trial	Takebe et al. (2015)
Enoticumab/ REGN421/ SAR153192	Solid tumor	Anti-DLL4	Under trial	Takebe et al. (2015)
Sonidegib	Pancreatic, breast cancer, medulloblastoma, solid tumors	HH (Hedgehog) signaling	Different stages of trials for different cancers	Takebe et al. (2015)

Table 1 Drugs Targeting CSCs/CSC Pathways in Clinical Trials—cont'd

Compound	Cancer Stem Cell	Mechanism	Clinical Trial	References
Glasdegib	Solid tumors, hematological malignancies	HH signaling	Phase I/II	Takebe et al. (2015)
PRI-724	Solid tumors, colorectal, pancreatic cancer, myeloid leukemia	CBP/beta-catenin antagonist	Under trial	Takebe et al. (2015)
LGK-974	Melanoma, breast, pancreatic cancer	Porcupine inhibitor	Under trial	Takebe et al. (2015)
Vantictumab/ OMP-18R5	Solid tumors	Antifrizzled-1/2/5/7/8 antibody	Under trial	Takebe et al. (2015)
OMP-54F28	Solid tumors	Antifrizzled 8-Fc decoy fusion protein	Under trial	Takebe et al. (2015)
OTSA101	Synovial sarcoma	Radiolabeled antifrizzled-10 antibody	Under trial	Takebe et al. (2015)

cells that replenish damaged tissues (Schmidt, 2012). But given their plasticity, even differentiated cells are capable of reverting back to a stem-like state after treatment, there is a pressing need for drug combinations and repeat treatments to eliminate CSCs in patients (Schmidt, 2012).

The effect of radiation has already been discussed in Section 1 of this review. Radiation leads to enrichment of CSCs as well as reprogramming of cells to acquire stem-like phenotypes. One approach to sensitize CSCs to radiation was through inhibition of Akt with the small molecule inhibitor perifosine, which led to a significant increase in apoptosis (Hambardzumyan et al., 2008). This strategy provides a rational means of potentially enhancing the efficacy of CSC therapy. However, these preclinical studies need to be supported by further translational studies to develop a clinically relevant, safe, and effective strategy for targeting death in CSCs.

2.2 Immunotherapy

ImmunoCellular Therapeutics, Ltd. is a company focused on developing immune-based therapies for the treatment of brain and other cancers. Their lead product candidate, ICT-107, a dendritic cell-based immunotherapy targeting multiple tumor-associated antigens on glioblastoma stem cells (Phuphanich et al., 2013), is currently in a Phase 3 clinical trial (information provided by the company website). ImmunoCellular's pipeline also includes ICT-121, a dendritic cell immunotherapy targeting the CD133 antigen on stem cells in recurrent glioblastoma; ICT-140, a dendritic cell immunotherapy targeting antigens on ovarian CSCs; and a Stem-to-T-cell research program which focuses on engineering the patient's own hematopoietic stem cells to generate antigen-specific cancer-killing T cells. Both ICT-140 and ICT-121 are currently in Phase 1 clinical trials (information provided by the company website). Studies have revealed that some chemotherapy drugs have the ability to activate an innate immune response in the tumor microenvironment through release of ligands for Toll-like and purinergic receptors that enable antitumor T-cell responses (Radvanyi, 2013). Studies have also shown that chemotherapeutic drug treatment (eg, cyclophosphamide) before immunotherapy is capable of transiently depleting CD4+ T-regulatory cells (Radvanyi, 2013). Additionally, recent clinical trials demonstrated that patients who received chemotherapy after immunotherapy showed much better responses and longer overall survival (Radvanyi, 2013). Immunotherapy may have assisted the increase of drug-sensitive subsets of tumor cells, or it could also be a result of chemotherapy-mediated increased sensitivity of the tumor cells to an ongoing memory T-cell response (Radvanyi, 2013). These studies emphasize the immediate need to study and carefully design more CSC-targeting immunotherapeutic trials.

2.3 Epigenetic Targeting

Epigenetic alterations are critical regulators of normal stem cell differentiation. The generation of CSCs may also involve parallel epigenetic reprogramming where loss of expression of differentiated state associated genes causes tumor cells to regain stem cell-specific features (Shukla & Meeran, 2014). DNA methylation, chromatin remodeling, and microRNA regulation are the possible modes of epigenetic regulation of CSCs (Shukla & Meeran, 2014) (Fig. 2). The oncogenic evolution of cancer stem and progenitor cells is partly orchestrated by dysregulated epigenetic mechanisms including aberrant DNA methylation leading to abnormal epigenetic memory (Shukla & Meeran, 2014). This might be the reason why epigenetic therapies that target DNA methyltransferases (DNMT) 1, DNMT3A, and

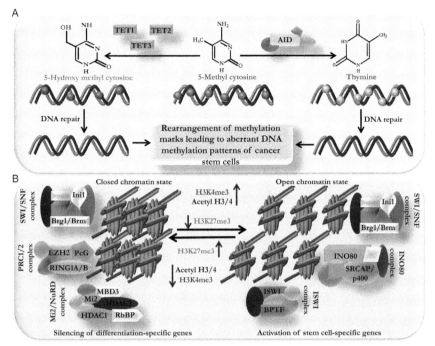

Fig. 2 The major signaling pathways associated with stemness in CSCs. *Reproduced with permission from Shukla, S., & Meeran, S. M. (2014). Epigenetics of cancer stem cells: Pathways and therapeutics.* Biochimica et Biophysica Acta, 1840, 3494–3502. (See the color plate.)

DNMT3B through 5-Azacitidine (Aza) and 5-Aza-2′-deoxycytidine (Aza-dC) have proven successful in the treatment of hematologic neoplasms (Wongtrakoongate, 2015). The DNMT inhibitor Aza is the first epigenetic drug approved by the Food and Drug Administration for treatment of myelodysplastic syndromes (MDS). Aza and Aza-dC can induce differentiation of Friend erythroleukemia cells (Wongtrakoongate, 2015). Recently, a failure of Aza to eradicate cancer stem and progenitor cells in patients with MDS and AML was reported (Wongtrakoongate, 2015). However, it is not clear if this indicates a need to improve the design of the Aza clinical trial, or to develop other improved drugs and combinatorial clinical schemes that can completely diminish the MDS and AML cancer stem and progenitor cells. Intriguingly, tranylcypromine, an inhibitor targeting histone H3 lysine 4 demethylase LSD1 a factor critical in AML stem maintenance showed promising results in combination with retinoic acid (RA) for the induction of AML myeloid differentiation (Wongtrakoongate, 2015). Treatment of medulloblastoma cell lines with Aza-dC has also shown interesting results

(Wongtrakoongate, 2015). Treatments with Aza and Aza-dC can lead to toxic side effects to hematopoietic, nervous as well as metabolic systems, however, these drugs are still less toxic as compared to traditional chemotherapy (Wongtrakoongate, 2015). Low-dose treatment with Aza-dC in patients with MDS and solid tumors lead to a complete response in patients, indicating that low-dose DNA methylation inhibitors may provide a safer therapeutic option especially for elderly and sensitive patients (Wongtrakoongate, 2015).

2.4 Differentiation Therapy

The ability to promote terminal differentiation in cancer cells reflects the plasticity of the differentiation program and transformed state in tumor cells (Leszczyniecka, Roberts, Dent, Grant, & Fisher, 2001; Staudt, Sarkar, & Fisher, 2007). This approach holds promise for cancer therapy, since agents used to promote terminal differentiation tend to be less toxic than conventional anticancer chemotherapeutic agents (Leszczyniecka et al., 2001; Staudt et al., 2007). Currently, numerous studies are focusing on the differentiation inducing potential of all-trans retinoic acids (ATRA), and because of the inherent stemness properties of CSCs, these cell types may be susceptible to differentiation therapies. Roughly 90% of acute promyelocytic leukemia (APL) patients attain complete remission and over 70% are cured by ATRA therapy with or without concomitant chemotherapy with methotrexate and cytarabine (Sell, 2004). The overall survival rate is markedly better in ATRA compared to chemotherapy alone and up to 75% disease-free 5-year survival rate is observed for both induction and maintenance on ATRA treatment (Sell, 2004). Acquired resistance to retinoid-induced maturation is still possible and this may be due to the fact that the mechanism of resistance to RA therapy is not well understood. The causal mechanisms may involve increased ATRA metabolism, increased expression of the RA-binding proteins, P-glycoprotein expression, or mutations in the ligand-binding domain of RAR-α (Marill, Idres, Capron, Nguyen, & Chabot, 2003). Combination strategies such as those involving other differentiating-inducing agents, histone deacetylase inhibitors, cytotoxic or chromatin-remodeling agents, as well as receptor-selective and modified retinoids may overcome this resistance (Sell, 2004). ATRA treatment also causes side effects, indicating dosing schedules are critical to the success of this treatment (Adès et al., 2010; Basma et al., 2016; Sell, 2004).

3. POTENTIAL THERAPEUTIC TARGETS AND STRATEGIES
3.1 Cell Surface Marker-Based Targeting

Although recent studies have expanded our appreciation of CSC surface molecules, the picture is far from complete. It is frequently observed that all CSCs do not express the same markers, or that normal cells also express similar surface antigens. CD133 (prominin-1) is a cell surface glycoprotein expressed on CSCs in several solid tumors such as glioma, lung, liver, and colorectal cancer and is responsible for a drug-resistant phenotype and poor prognosis (Dragu, Necula, Bleotu, Diaconu, & Chivu-Economescu, 2015). For this reason, several strategies for anti-CD133 therapy have been developed. However, CD133 expression is not restricted to CSCs and some CD133 negative cancer cells can also initiate cancer (eg, colon cancer and glioblastoma). CD44, a transmembrane protein regulating cell adhesion by acting as a receptor for hyaluronic acid, selectin, collagen, osteopontin, fibronectin, and laminin, is another important marker for several CSC types. Antihuman CD44 monoclonal antibody treatment is reported to induce myeloid differentiation in patient-derived AML blasts, inhibit homing to the microenvironmental niche, and alter stem cell fate (Jin, Hope, Zhai, Smadja-Joffe, & Dick, 2006). When combined with doxorubicin and cyclophosphamide it prevented relapse of aggressive breast cancer (Dragu et al., 2015). In pancreatic cancer, a mouse IgG1 antihuman CD44 receptor decreased in vitro tumor sphere formation and inhibited pancreatic tumor growth, metastasis, and tumor recurrence (Dragu et al., 2015). Similar results were obtained in breast, lung, bladder, larynx, and colorectal cancers (Dragu et al., 2015). CD47, a transmembrane protein receptor for thrombospondin family members and for signal regulatory protein alpha (SIRPα), is widely expressed on AML CSCs and other solid tumors (Dragu et al., 2015). Two anti-CD47 mAbs such as B6H12.2 and B6H12 were developed as a strategy for cancer therapy and promising results were obtained in AML, glioblastoma, and ovarian, breast, colon, and bladder cancer, and non-Hodgkin lymphoma, acute lymphoblastic leukemia and multiple myeloma CSCs (Dragu et al., 2015). There are other FDA-approved antibodies for the treatment of solid and hematological tumors, such as rituximab (anti-CD20), cetuximab (anti-EGFR), trastuzumab (anti-HER2), bevacizumab (anti-VEGF-A), ipilimumab (anti-CTLA-4), and pembrolizumab (anti-PD-1) that are currently used for immunotherapy against tumor cells and may also prove helpful against CSCs (Dragu et al., 2015).

3.2 Molecular Marker-Based Targeting

3.2.1 MDA-9/Syntenin (SDCBP)

Melanoma differentiation associated gene-9/Syntenin (MDA-9/Syntenin; syndecan binding protein (SDCBP)) is a scaffold protein, which regulates tumor pathogenesis in multiple cancers (Boukerche et al., 2005; Das et al., 2012; Kegelman et al., 2014, 2015; Qian et al., 2013; Sarkar, Boukerche, Su, & Fisher, 2008). MDA-9 interacts with a wide range of key regulatory proteins, including SRC, FAK, and EGFR, which are often coupled with expression of the tumor phenotype and cancer progression (Kegelman et al., 2014; Sarkar et al., 2008). MDA-9 is a diagnostic marker of tumor aggression and grade in gliomas, melanomas, and breast cancer (Boukerche et al., 2005; Das et al., 2012; Kegelman et al., 2014, 2015; Qian et al., 2013; Sarkar et al., 2008). Elevated MDA-9 levels also correspond with poor prognosis (Kegelman et al., 2014). Bioinformatics analysis has shown the possible interaction of MDA-9 with STAT3, C-Myc, NANOG, OCT4, and SOX2 (Bacolod et al., 2015) (Fig. 3). Highly aggressive cancers which express elevated levels of MDA-9 are also observed to contain increased populations of CSCs. MDA-9 has recently been shown to facilitate cancer stemness and survival (unpublished observation). Mechanistically, MDA-9 regulates multiple stemness genes (*Nanog, Oct4,* and *Sox2*) through activation of STAT3. MDA-9 controls survival of CSCs by activating the NOTCH1 pathway through phospho-Src and DLL1. Once activated, cleaved NOTCH1 directs c-Myc expression through RBPJK thereby facilitating CSC growth and proliferation. Knockdown of MDA-9 affected the NOTCH1/C-Myc and p-STAT3/*Nanog* pathways causing a loss of stemness and initiation of apoptosis. A clear association between stemness and MDA-9 expression was evident in GBM, prostate, and breast cancer as well as in normal astrocytes, and normal prostate and breast epithelial cells (unpublished observation). A positive influence of MDA-9 on CSC survival, growth, and angiogenesis was also observed. MDA-9 promoted stem cell phenotypes and survival through regulation of NOTCH1, C-Myc, STAT3, and *Nanog* in GBM, prostate, and breast CSCs. Indications of possible chemoresistance regulation was indicated by the correlative expression of Axl and MDA-9. This previously unidentified relationship between MDA-9 and CSCs, on multiple molecular levels, emphasizes the significance of this gene as a potential new exciting therapeutic target. CD133 a proneural GBM CSC and poor prognosis marker, as wells as CD44, a characteristic marker for mesenchymal GBM CSCs (Brown et al., 2015; Mao et al., 2013; Wang et al., 2009) were both significantly down-regulated post *mda-9* knock-down (unpublished observation). These results

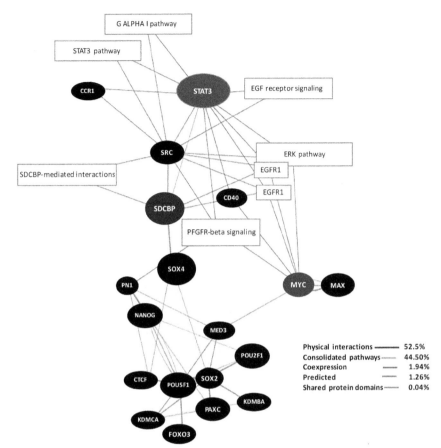

Fig. 3 Schematic representation of bioinformatics analysis predicting the possible interaction of MDA-9/Syntenin (SDCBP) with STAT3, C-Myc, NANOG, OCT4, and SOX2. (See the color plate.)

indicate the efficacy of MDA-9 in regulation of CSCs at multiple levels (Fig. 4), suggesting it's potential as an appropriate target for CSC therapy.

3.2.2 Transporters

Even though in vivo tumors as well as CSCs express functional ABC transporters, attempts at reversing MDR have not proven very successful. ABC transport inhibitors need to be repurposed as "CSC sensitizers" as they might not reduce tumor burden immediately; however, their effectiveness may be quantified using alternative endpoints, such as the frequency of relapse or the time to relapse (Dean, 2009). In such scenarios, it will be important to develop a panel of ABC transporter inhibitors, involving ABCG2 which is one of the most important transporters for stem cells (Dean, 2009). Some

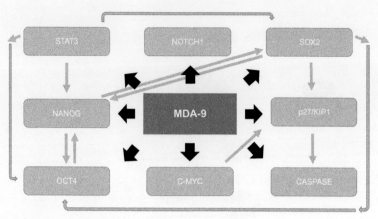

Fig. 4 Schematic representation of the multiple levels of CSC regulation by MDA-9/Syntenin(SDCBP). (See the color plate.)

ABCG2 inhibitors such as fumitremorgin C (FTC) and Ko143 are specific to ABCG2; however, they are toxic to cells and mice (Dean, 2009). Studies on ABCG2 inhibitors has generated a set of new contenders such as peptides mimicking transmembrane domains of ABC transporters, which have proven to be selective and specific inhibitors, and in principle could be developed for any transporter (Dean, 2009). GF120918 and other ABCB1 inhibitors are also known to be effective against ABCG2 (Dean, 2009; Lou & Dean, 2007), indicating that other pan–ABC inhibitors may also have potential applications for targeting ABCG2. The combined use of chemotherapeutic drugs and inhibitors targeting ABC transporters could be employed to selectively and more efficiently kill CSCs (Dean, 2009). However, complete eradication of CSCs by this method may be hard to achieve in vivo without concomitant toxicity and the death of normal stem cells, particularly those of the bone marrow. Furthermore, both ABCG2 and ABCB1 play an important role in maintaining the blood–brain barrier (Lou & Dean, 2007). Designing a "therapeutic window" strategy that destroys the CSCs, but spares normal stem cells is required (Dean, 2009).

3.2.3 PTCH Pathway
Another potential strategy to restrict CSC development and maintenance could be targeting the parallel pathways essential for the growth and maintenance of normal stem cells. The PTCH/HH pathway could be one such potential target, which is comprised of several genes that can act as either tumor suppressor genes or oncogenes, and is often dysregulated in stem cell activation in cancers (Dean, 1997, 2006). PTCH is the receptor for HH molecules and the *PTCH* gene is mutated in patients with inherited

disorders including nevoid basal cell carcinoma syndrome, spontaneous basal cell carcinomas as well as some medulloblastomas, rhabdomyomas, and rhabdomyosarcomas (Lou & Dean, 2007). Due to the prevalence of the *PTCH* gene in cancers, it is not surprising that the mammalian *HH* genes are also overexpressed in many cancer cell lines derived from small cell lung, pancreatic, gastric, breast, and prostate cancers (Lou & Dean, 2007).

Cyclopamine is a steroid-like compound that can inhibit the growth of cells and tumors with activated HH signaling (Lou & Dean, 2007). Recently, it has been reported that vitamin D3 is an important molecule in PTCH signaling. Vitamin D3 and/or other steroidal analogs could also be considered for CSC targeting; however, detailed expression analysis of the mRNA or protein of these genes would be useful for evaluating the effectiveness of this targeted therapy (Lou & Dean, 2007).

3.3 Epigenetic Targeting

Aza- and Aza-dC-based epigenetic treatments have been successful and this spurred many researchers to use these agents to target CSCs in different types of cancer. Studies have also focused on the differentiation promoting abilities of Aza-dC in different CSCs. Aza-dC has recently been reported to induce expression of microRNA-137, which is involved in inhibiting proliferation and modulating differentiation of glioblastoma stem cells (Wongtrakoongate, 2015). Promising results have been obtained in prostate and pancreatic CSCs, where this treatment decreased tumor proliferation, decreased expression of stemness genes, and induced differentiation of CSCs (Wongtrakoongate, 2015). Detailed long-term studies need to be performed to ascertain whether low-dose Aza or Aza-dC treatments could alter the fates of stem and progenitor cells without side effects and toxicity in patients (Wongtrakoongate, 2015). Apart from Aza treatment, studies are also focused on the importance of DNA methylation on CSC regulation among which DNMT1, DNMT3a, and DNMT3b are potential therapeutic targets (Shukla & Meeran, 2014). Studies demonstrated that the polycomb group of proteins (PcG) were more prone to hypermethylation in CSCs than in embryonic stem cells. Differential hypermethylation as well as hypomethylation results have been observed in CSCs, which were correlated with poor prognosis (Shukla & Meeran, 2014). Strategies centering on appropriate methylation targets might prove important in controlling stemness as well as eliminating CSCs. Chromatin remodeling is also an important epigenetic regulatory mechanism of CSCs (Shukla & Meeran, 2014). Brahma-related gene 1 (BRG1), is a possible potential target by the virtue of its ability to epigenetically regulate the Wnt pathway, repressing pluripotency gene targets, OCT4 and SOX2, and inhibiting tumor-initiating cell populations (Shukla & Meeran, 2014). Polycomb repressive complex have been studied by many groups and their importance as a CSC target is also well studied (Shukla & Meeran, 2014). Other remodeling complexes important for CSC regulation and maintenance are ISWI complex, CHD, and INO80 remodeling complexes (Shukla & Meeran, 2014). Addressing these epigenetic targets will not only provide an understanding of CSC biology but will also shed light on development of potential novel clinical regimens (Wongtrakoongate, 2015).

3.4 ncRNA-Based Targeting

The relevance of noncoding RNAs (ncRNA) in human cancer is receiving increased attention. ncRNAs can be broadly classified based on their transcript size into small ncRNAs (less than 200 nucleotides, consisting of miRNAs, siRNAs, piRNAs, and tiRNAs) and long ncRNAs (lncRNAs, longer than 200 nucleotides); snoRNAs are intermediate in size, 60–300 bp (Huang, Alvarez, Hu, & Cheng, 2013). The involvement of ncRNAs in human cancers is particularly significant for microRNAs (miRNAs) and long noncoding RNAs (lncRNAs). miRNAs have been extensively studied for their roles in cancers, and lncRNAs are currently coming to light as important mediators in the cancer paradigm (Huang et al., 2013). These ncRNAs are frequently dysregulated in a variety of human cancers, but their biological functions still remain largely unknown. Recently, studies have reported dysregulated ncRNAs in CSCs (Huang et al., 2013). miRNAs comprise a major factor in the regulation of stem cells and in CSCs. LIN28 miRNA inhibits the tumor suppressor activity and regulates ALDH1, a marker for CSCs (Charafe-Jauffret et al., 2010; Yang et al., 2010). miRNA expression profile analysis of embryonic stem cells and breast CSCs revealed an overlap, with 37 miRNAs differentially expressed in CD44+CD24−/-low breast CSCs, especially three clusters of miR-200 family miRNAs, miR-200c-141, miR-200b-200a-429, and miR-183-96-182 (Shimono et al., 2009). This differential expression of miRNAs was also observed in colon CSCs (Huang et al., 2013). Several studies determined the role of miRNAs in CSC regulation and maintenance. miR-22 is reported to suppress the expression of miR-200 family members in breast CSCs by regulating chromatin-remodeling enzymes leading to induction of EMT and stemness in breast CSCs (Song et al., 2013). miR-128 is reported to decrease the self-renewal capacity of CSCs via BMI, miR-125 promoted cell proliferation by regulating CDK6 and CDC25, miR-181 regulated differentiation by targeting transcription factors CDX2 and GATA6 (Huang et al., 2013). In pancreatic CSCs a signature of 210 miRNAs regulating self-renewal and differentiation was observed including miR-99a, miR-100, miR-125b, miR-192, and miR-429, while miR-34 was shown to be downregulated (Huang et al., 2013). The importance of miR-34 was also apparent in gastric cancer cells, where it was able to attenuate stemness-associated genes like NOTCH (Ji et al., 2008). miRNA mimics and lentiviral-expressed miRNAs may have significant potential in restoring tumor suppressor miRNAs in CSCs (Huang et al., 2013). In comparison to extensively studied miRNA, lncRNAs have just begun to be incorporated into therapeutic strategies against cancer; however, they also hold promise as potential targets. lncRNAs are often dysregulated in cancer and they also play critical roles in regulating pluripotency in embryonic stem cells and considering these functions they could also target CSCs by regulating similar pathways and molecules such as OCT4, SOX2, KLF4, and PcG (Eades et al., 2014). Another potential function of lncRNAs could be to competitively inhibit miRNAs by serving as a negative molecular sponge targeting CSC maintenance gene functions (Eades et al., 2014). Investigative studies focusing on the different functions of ncRNAs in CSCs may assist in the design of new therapeutic targets and mechanisms for overcoming chemoresistance.

3.5 Differentiation Therapy

The underlying premise of differentiation therapy is that tumor cells can be reprogrammed to differentiate and to cease proliferation, thereby controlling their tumorigenic and malignant potential (Leszczyniecka et al., 2001; Staudt et al., 2007). Although a number of agents have been studied over the years, the most thoroughly examined and clinically tested as a differentiating agent is RA (Vitamin A), in particular ATRA. RA-induced differentiation therapy has acquired a therapeutic niche in treatment of APL and the ability of RA to prevent cancer and induce differentiation is currently being investigated (Gudas & Wagner, 2011; Karsy, Albert, Tobias, Murali, & Jhanwar-Uniyal, 2010; Sell, 2004). Salinomycin is reported to induce expression of the epithelial/MET marker E-cadherin in these tumors, indicating that salinomycin might eradicate CSCs by inducing their differentiation (Beug, 2009). CD105+ renal CSCs treated with rhIL-15 were observed to undergo epithelial differentiation of all CD105+ CSC subsets and blocked CSC self-renewal and their tumorigenic properties in severe combined immunodeficient mice (Azzi et al., 2011).

3.6 Immunotherapy

Immunotherapy also holds great promise in the elimination of circulating and noncirculating CSCs. Natural killer cells and γδ T cells were studied to design innate immune responders against CSCs. In vitro CSC-primed T cells have shown success in targeting CSCs in vivo after adoptive transfer (Pan et al., 2015). A CSC-based dendritic cell vaccine resulted in significant induction of anti-CSC immunity both in vitro and in vivo (Pan et al., 2015). Identification of specific antigens or genetic alterations in CSCs such as ALDH, CD44, CD133, and HER2 may serve as useful targets for CSC immunotherapy (Pan et al., 2015). Due to the dependence of CSCs on the CSC niche, these interactions may serve as additional targets for CSC immunotherapy, such as interrupting interactions of myeloid-derived suppressor cells; signaling molecules, such as IL-6 and IL-8; and immune checkpoint inhibitors, such as PD-1/PD-L1 (Pan et al., 2015). Recent studies have reported that a subset of drug-resistant cells in subcutaneous tumors that overexpressed TOPO-IIα could be selectively eradicated using doxorubicin (Radvanyi, 2013). Other studies also support the power of combining immunotherapy with chemotherapy, and that immunotherapy may reveal new strategies although ineffective by themselves, in combination they can effectively target CSCs. Recent studies also suggest that an adaptive cancer vaccination approach in which multiple cDNA vaccines can be made at different times can be utilized as a personalized therapy for individual patients (Radvanyi, 2013).

4. CONCLUSIONS AND FUTURE PERSPECTIVES

CSCs are constantly evolving, functionally heterogeneous cells that are nurtured by the plasticity of its niche. In spite of increased interest and research in this field, our understanding of cellular and molecular mechanisms that underlie CSC properties is still very limited. To date, chemotherapy and radiotherapy represent the two major options for cancer treatment; however, CSCs are often resistant to these treatments. Evasion of anoikis and immune surveillance, quiescence and plasticity of the CSC niche add further challenges to the eradication of CSCs. Combination therapy and therapeutic strategies based on detailed understanding of the CSC niche would assist greatly in developing approaches for targeting CSCs. Detailed studies will enable us to potentially discover new clinically effective targets that are yet unknown. Considering the tremendous role of CSCs and distinct dysregulation of many interconnected pathways, researchers are currently trying to design appropriate responses to provide novel strategies for future cancer therapy. CSCs are challenging medical problems and defining appropriate therapeutic targets and strategies to attack these targets are urgently needed to alter this cancer paradigm and enhance therapy. Researchers should view each challenge as a window of opportunity to delve into this intriguing subpopulation of cancer cells.

This review discusses some of the therapeutic strategies that are currently in the pipeline, and some potential targets for CSC therapy. This is clearly an evolving field of research and more than incremental results can be anticipated in the not too distant future. Molecular targets that regulate CSCs on multiple levels, maintain/disrupt therapy resistance, and induce immune sensitivity and differentiation have potential to lead to the development of future drugs that are capable of clinically eradicating and preventing the generation of new CSCs in patients. These drugs would in principle provide a means of preventing metastasis and relapse, reducing morbidity and toxicity, and provide beneficial enduring outcomes in cancer patients.

ACKNOWLEDGMENTS

Support for our laboratories was provided in part by National Institutes of Health Grants R01 CA097318 (P.B.F.), R01 CA168517 (Maurizio Pellecchia and P.B.F.), and P50 CA058326 (Martin G. Pomper and P.B.F.); the Samuel Waxman Cancer Research Foundation (P.B.F. and D.S.); National Foundation for Cancer Research (P.B.F.); NCI Cancer Center Support Grant to VCU Massey Cancer Center P30 CA016059 (P.B.F. and D.S.); and VCU Massey Cancer Center developmental funds (P.B.F.). D.S. is the Harrison Foundation Distinguished Professor in Cancer Research in the VCU Massey Cancer Center. P.B.F. and D.S. are SWCRF Investigators. P.B.F. holds the Thelma Newmeyer Corman Chair in Cancer Research in the VCU Massey Cancer Center.

Conflict of Interest: Dr. Paul B. Fisher is a cofounder of, serves as a consultant to and has ownership interest in Cancer Targeting Systems (CTS), Inc. Johns Hopkins University, Virginia Commonwealth University, and Columbia University have ownership interest in CTS, Inc.

REFERENCES

Adès, L., Guerci, A., Raffoux, E., Sanz, M., Chevallier, P., Lapusan, S., et al. (2010). Very long-term outcome of acute promyelocytic leukemia after treatment with all-trans retinoic acid and chemotherapy: The European APL Group experience. *Blood*, *115*, 1690–1696.

Ailles, L. E., & Weissman, I. L. (2007). Cancer stem cells in solid tumors. *Curent Opinion in Biotechnology*, *18*, 460–466.

Allan, A. L., Vantyghem, S. A., Tuck, A. B., & Chambers, A. F. (2006). Tumor dormancy and cancer stem cells: Implications for the biology and treatment of breast cancer metastasis. *Breast Disease*, *26*, 87–98.

Azzi, S., Bruno, S., Giron-Michel, J., Clay, D., Devocelle, A., Croce, M., et al. (2011). Differentiation therapy: Targeting human renal cancer stem cells with interleukin 15. *Journal of National Cancer Institute, 103*, 1884–1898.

Baccelli, I., & Trumpp, A. (2012). The evolving concept of cancer and metastasis stem cells. *The Journal of Cell Biology, 198*, 281–293.

Bacolod, M. D., Das, S. K., Sokhi, U. K., Bradley, S., Fenstermacher, D. A., Pellecchia, M., et al. (2015). Examination of epigenetic and other molecular factors associated with mda-9/syntenin dysregulation in cancer through integrated analyses of public genomic datasets. *Advances in Cancer Research, 127*, 49–121.

Balbous, A., Cortes, U., Guilloteau, K., Villalva, C., Flamant, S., Gaillard, A., et al. (2014). A mesenchymal glioma stem cell profile is related to clinical outcome. *Oncogenesis, 3*, e91.

Bao, S., Wu, Q., McLendon, R. E., Hao, Y., Shi, Q., Hjelmeland, A. B., et al. (2006). Glioma stem cells promote radioresistance by preferential activation of the DNA damage response. *Nature, 444*, 756–760.

Basma, H., Ghayad, S. E., Rammal, G., Mancinelli, A., Harajly, M., Ghamloush, F., et al. (2016). The synthetic retinoid ST1926 as a novel therapeutic agent in rhabdomyosarcoma. *International Journal of Cancer, 138*, 1528–1537.

Besançon, R., Valsesia-Wittmann, S., Puisieux, A., Caron de Fromentel, C., & Maguer-Satta, V. (2009). Cancer stem cells: The emerging challenge of drug targeting. *Current Medicinal Chemistry, 16*, 394–416.

Beug, H. (2009). Breast cancer stem cells: Eradication by differentiation therapy? *Cell, 138*, 623–625.

Bhat-Nakshatri, P., Goswami, C. P., Badve, S., Sledge, G. W., Jr., & Nakshatri, H. (2013). Identification of FDA-approved drugs targeting breast cancer stem cells along with biomarkers of sensitivity. *Scientific Reports, 3*, 2530.

Bjerkvig, R., Tysnes, B. B., Aboody, K. S., Najbauer, J., & Terzis, A. J. (2005). Opinion: The origin of the cancer stem cell: Current controversies and new insights. *Nature Reviews. Cancer, 5*, 899–904.

Boukerche, H., Su, Z. Z., Emdad, L., Baril, P., Balme, B., Thomas, L., et al. (2005). mda-9/Syntenin: A positive regulator of melanoma metastasis. *Cancer Research, 65*, 10901–10911.

Brown, D. V., Daniel, P. M., D'Abaco, G. M., Gogos, A., Ng, W., Morokoff, A. P., et al. (2015). Coexpression analysis of CD133 and CD44 identifies proneural and mesenchymal subtypes of glioblastoma multiforme. *Oncotarget, 6*, 6267–6280.

Bruttel, V. S., & Wischhusen, J. (2014). Cancer stem cell immunology: Key to understanding tumorigenesis and tumor immune escape? *Frontiers in Immunology, 5*, 360.

Cabrera, M. C., Hollingsworth, R. E., & Hurt, E. M. (2015). Cancer stem cell plasticity and tumor hierarchy. *World Journal of Stem Cells, 7*, 27–36.

Charafe-Jauffret, E., Ginestier, C., Iovino, F., Tarpin, C., Diebel, M., Esterni, B., et al. (2010). Aldehyde dehydrogenase 1-positive cancer stem cells mediate metastasis and poor clinical outcome in inflammatory breast cancer. *Clinical Cancer Research, 16*, 45–55.

Cojoc, M. C., Peitzsch, I., Kurth, F., Trautmann, L. A., Kunz-Schughart, G. D., Telegeev, E. A., et al. (2015). Aldehyde dehydrogenase is regulated by beta-catenin/TCF and promotes radioresistance in prostate cancer progenitor cells. *Cancer Research, 75*, 1482–1494.

Crowley, E., McDevitt, C. A., & Callaghan, R. (2010). Generating inhibitors of P-glycoprotein: Where to, now? *Methods in Molecular Biology, 596*, 405–432.

Dakubo, G. D., Jakupciak, J. P., Birch-Machin, M. A., & Parr, R. L. (2007). Clinical implications and utility of field cancerization. *Cancer Cell International, 7*, 2.

Das, S. K., Bhutia, S. K., Sokhi, U. K., Azab, B., Su, Z. Z., Boukerche, H., et al. (2012). Raf kinase inhibitor RKIP inhibits MDA-9/syntenin-mediated metastasis in melanoma. *Cancer Research, 72*, 6217–6226.

Dean, M. (1997). Towards a unified model of tumor suppression: Lessons learned from the human patched gene. *Biochimica et Biophysica Acta, 1332,* M43–M52.

Dean, M. (2006). Cancer stem cells: Redefining the paradigm of cancer treatment strategies. *Molecular Interventions, 6,* 140–148.

Dean, M. (2009). ABC transporters, drug resistance, and cancer stem cells. *Journal of Mammary Gland Biology and Neoplasia, 14,* 3–9.

Doyle, L. A., Yang, W., Abruzzo, L. V., Krogmann, T., Gao, Y., Rishi, A. K., et al. (1998). A multidrug resistance transporter from human MCF-7 breast cancer cells. *Proceedings of the National Academy of Sciences of the United States of America, 95,* 15665–15670.

Dragu, D. L., Necula, L. G., Bleotu, C., Diaconu, C. C., & Chivu-Economescu, M. (2015). Therapies targeting cancer stem cells: Current trends and future challenges. *World Journal of Stem Cells, 7,* 1185–1201.

Eades, G., Zhang, Y.-S., Li, Q.-L., Xia, J.-X., Yao, Y., & Zhou, Q. (2014). Long noncoding RNAs in stem cells and cancer. *World Journal of Clinical Oncology, 5,* 134–141.

Enderling, H. (2013). Cancer stem cells and tumor dormancy. *Advances in Experimental Medicine and Biology, 734,* 55–71.

Fang, L., Zhu, Q., Neuenschwander, M., Specker, E., Wulf-Goldenberg, A., Weis, W. I., et al. (2016). A small-molecule antagonist of the β-catenin/TCF4 interaction blocks the self-renewal of cancer stem cells and suppresses tumorigenesis. *Cancer Research, 76,* 801–901.

Fofaria, N. M., & Srivastava, S. K. (2015). STAT3 induces anoikis resistance, promotes cell invasion and metastatic potential in pancreatic cancer cells. *Carcinogenesis, 36,* 142–150.

Frisch, S. M., Schaller, M., & Cieply, B. (2013). Mechanisms that link the oncogenic epithelial-mesenchymal transition to suppression of anoikis. *Journal of Cell Science, 126,* 21–29.

Ghajar, C. M. (2015). Metastasis prevention by targeting the dormant niche. *Nature Reviews. Cancer, 15,* 238–247.

Giancotti, F. G. (2013). Mechanisms governing metastatic dormancy and reactivation. *Cell, 155,* 750–764.

Gudas, L. J., & Wagner, J. A. (2011). Retinoids regulate stem cell differentiation. *Journal of Cellular Physiology, 226,* 322–330.

Hambardzumyan, D., Becher, O. J., Rosenblum, M. K., Pandolfi, P. P., Manova-Todorova, K., & Holland, E. C. (2008). PI3K pathway regulates survival of cancer stem cells residing in the perivascular niche following radiation in medullolastoma *in vivo. Genes and Development, 22,* 436–448.

Huang, T., Alvarez, A., Hu, B., & Cheng, S.-Y. (2013). Noncoding RNAs in cancer and cancer stem cells. *Chinese Journal of Cancer, 32,* 582–593.

Ji, Q., Hao, X., Meng, Y., Zhang, M., Desano, J., Fan, D., et al. (2008). Restoration of tumor suppressor miR-34 inhibits human p53-mutant gastric cancer tumorspheres. *BMC Cancer, 8,* 266.

Ji, J., & Wang, X. W. (2012). Clinical implications of cancer stem cell biology in hepatocellular carcinoma. *Seminars in Oncology, 39,* 461–472.

Jin, L., Hope, K. J., Zhai, Q., Smadja-Joffe, F., & Dick, J. E. (2006). Targeting of CD44 eradicates human acute myeloid leukemic stem cells. *Nature Medicine, 12,* 1167–1174.

Kantara, C., O'Connell, M. R., Luthra, G., Gajjar, A., Sarkar, S., Ullrich, R. L., et al. (2015). Methods for detecting circulating cancer stem cells (CCSCs) as a novel approach for diagnosis of colon cancer relapse/metastasis. *Laboratory Investigation, 95,* 100–112.

Karsy, M., Albert, L., Tobias, M. E., Murali, R., & Jhanwar-Uniyal, M. (2010). All-trans retinoic acid modulates cancer stem cells of glioblastoma multiforme in an MAPK-dependent manner. *Anticancer Research, 30,* 4915–4920.

Katoh, S., Goi, T., Naruse, T., Ueda, Y., Kurebayashi, H., Nakazawa, T., et al. (2015). Cancer stem cell marker in circulating tumor cells: Expression of CD44 variant exon

9 is strongly correlated to treatment refractoriness, recurrence and prognosis of human colorectal cancer. *Anticancer Research, 35,* 239–244.

Kawasaki, B. T., & Farrar, W. L. (2008). Cancer stem cells, CD200 and immunoevasion. *Trends in Immunology, 29,* 464–468.

Kegelman, T. P., Das, S. K., Emdad, L., Hu, B., Menezes, M. E., Bhoopathi, P., et al. (2015). Targeting tumor invasion: The roles of MDA-9/Syntenin. *Expert Opinion on Therapeutic Targets, 19,* 97–112.

Kegelman, T. P., Das, S. K., Hu, B., Bacolod, M. D., Fuller, C. E., Menezes, M. E., et al. (2014). MDA-9/syntenin is a key regulator of glioma pathogenesis. *Neuro-oncology, 16,* 50–61.

Kim, H. (2015). Clinical implication of colorectal cancer stem cells: Still has a long way to go. *Annals of Coloproctology, 3,* 179–180.

Kim, Y. N., Koo, K. H., Sung, J. Y., Yun, U. J., & Kim, H. (2012). Anoikis resistance: An essential prerequisite for tumor metastasis. *International Journal of Cell Biology, 2012,* 306879.

Kleffel, S., & Schatton, T. (2013). Tumor dormancy and cancer stem cells: Two sides of the same coin? *Advances in Experimental Medicine and Biology, 734,* 145–179.

Kolev, V. N., Wright, Q. G., Vidal, C. M., Ring, J. E., Shapiro, I. M., Ricono, J., et al. (2015). PI3K/mTOR dual inhibitor VS-5584 preferentially targets cancer stem cells. *Cancer Research, 75,* 446–455.

Krause, M., Dubrovska, A., Linge, A., & Baumann, M. (2016). Cancer stem cells: Radioresistance, prediction of radiotherapy outcome and specific targets for combined treatments. *Advanced Drug Delivery Reviews.* pii: S0169-409X(16)30052-7. doi: 10.1016/j.addr.2016.02.002. [Epub ahead of print].

Kreso, A., & Dick, J. E. (2014). Evolution of the cancer stem cell model. *Cell Stem Cell, 14,* 275–291.

Kruyt, F. A., & Schuringa, J. J. (2010). Apoptosis and cancer stem cells: Implications for apoptosis targeted therapy. *Biochemical Pharmacology, 80,* 423–430.

Kurth, I., Hein, L., Mäbert, K., Peitzsch, C., Koi, L., Cojoc, M., et al. (2015). Cancer stem cell related markers of radioresistance in head and neck squamous cell carcinoma. *Oncotarget, 6,* 34494–34509.

Lagadec, C., Vlashi, E., Della Donna, L., Dekmezian, C., & Pajonk, F. (2012). Radiation-induced reprogramming of breast cancer cells. *Stem Cells, 30,* 833–844.

Leon, G., MacDonagh, L., Finn, S. P., Cuffe, S., & Barr, M. P. (2016). Cancer stem cells in drug resistant lung cancer: Targeting cell surface markers and signaling pathways. *Pharmacology & Therapeutics, 158,* 71–90.

Leszczyniecka, M., Roberts, T., Dent, P., Grant, S., & Fisher, P. B. (2001). Differentiation therapy of cancer: Basic science and clinical applications. *Pharmacology & Therapeutics, 90,* 105–156.

Liu, R., Wang, X., Chen, G. Y., Dalerba, P., Gurney, A., Hoey, T., et al. (2007). The prognostic role of a gene signature from tumorigenic breast-cancer cells. *The New England Journal of Medicine, 356,* 217–226.

Lou, H., & Dean, M. (2007). Targeted therapy for cancer stem cells: The patched pathway and ABC transporters. *Oncogene, 26,* 1357–1360.

Lv, J., & Shim, J. S. (2015). Existing drugs and their application in drug discovery targeting cancer stem cells. *Archives of Pharmacal Research, 38,* 1617–1626.

Mao, P., Joshi, K., Li, J., Kim, S. H., Li, P., Santana-Santos, L., et al. (2013). Mesenchymal glioma stem cells are maintained by activated glycolytic metabolism involving aldehyde dehydrogenase 1A3. *Proceedings of the National Academy of Sciences of the Unites States of America, 110,* 8644–8649.

Marill, J., Idres, N., Capron, C. C., Nguyen, E., & Chabot, G. G. (2003). Retinoic acid metabolism and mechanism of action: A review. *Current Drug Metabolism, 4,* 1–10.

Mathieu, J., Zhang, Z., Zhou, W., Wang, A. J., Heddleston, J. M., Pinna, C. M., et al. (2011). HIF induces human embryonic stem cell markers in cancer cells. *Cancer Research*, *71*, 4640–4652.

McInnes, L. M., Jacobson, N., Redfern, A., Dowling, A., Thompson, E. W., & Saunders, C. M. (2015). Clinical implications of circulating tumor cells of breast cancer patients: Role of epithelial–mesenchymal plasticity. *Frontiers in Oncology*, *5*, 42.

Nahas, G. R., Patel, S. A., Bliss, S. A., & Rameshwar, P. (2012). Can breast cancer stem cells evade the immune system? *Current Medicinal Chemistry*, *19*, 6036–6049.

Noh, K. H., Kim, B. W., Song, K. H., Cho, H., Lee, Y. H., Kim, J. H., et al. (2012). Nanog signaling in cancer promotes stem-like phenotype and immune evasion. *Journal of Clinical Investigation*, *122*, 4077–4093.

Obenauf, A. C., & Massagué, J. (2015). Surviving at a distance: Organ specific metastasis. *Trends in Cancer*, *1*, 76–91.

Oskarsson, T., & Massagué, J. (2012). Extracellular matrix players in metastatic niches. *EMBO Journal*, *31*, 254–256.

Pachter, J. A., Kolev, V. N., Schunselaar, L., Shapiro, I. M., Bueno, R., Baas, P., et al. (2015). FAK inhibitor VS-6063 (defactinib) targets mesothelioma cancer stem cells, which are enriched by standard of care chemotherapy. *Cancer Research*, *75*, 4236.

Pajonk, F., & Vlashi, E. (2013). Characterization of the stem cell niche and its importance in radiobiological response. *Seminars in Radiation Oncology*, *23*, 237–241.

Pajonk, F., Vlashi, E., & McBride, W. H. (2010). Radiation resistance of cancer stem cells: The 4 R's of radiobiology revisited. *Stem Cells*, *28*, 639–648.

Pallini, R., Ricci-Vitiani, L., Banna, G. L., Signore, M., Lombardi, D., Todaro, M., et al. (2008). Cancer stem cell analysis and clinical outcome in patients with glioblastoma multiforme. *Clinical Cancer Research*, *14*, 8205–8212.

Pan, Q., Li, Q., Liu, S., Ning, N., Zhang, X., Xu, Y., et al. (2015). Targeting cancer stem cells using immunologic approaches. *Stem Cells*, *33*, 2085–2092.

Patel, P., & Chen, E. I. (2012). Cancer stem cells, tumor dormancy, and metastasis. *Frontiers in Endocrinology*, *3*, 125.

Phuphanich, S., Wheeler, C. J., Rudnick, J. D., Mazer, M., Wang, H., Nuño, M. A., et al. (2013). Phase I trial of a multi-epitope-pulsed dendritic cell vaccine for patients with newly diagnosed glioblastoma. *Cancer Immunology, Immunotherapy*, *62*, 125–135.

Qian, X. L., Li, Y. Q., Yu, B., Gu, F., Liu, F. F., Li, W. D., et al. (2013). Syndecan binding protein (SDCBP) is overexpressed in estrogen receptor negative breast cancers, and is a potential promoter for tumor proliferation. *PLoS One*, *8*, e60046.

Radvanyi, L. (2013). Immunotherapy exposes cancer stem cell resistance and a new synthetic lethality. *Molecular Therapy*, *21*, 1472–1474.

Rich, J. N. (2007). Cancer stem cells in radiation resistance. *Cancer Research*, *67*, 8980–8984.

Roninson, I. B., Chin, J. E., Choi, K. G., Gros, P., Housman, D. E., Fojo, A., et al. (1986). Isolation of human mdr DNA sequences amplified in multidrug-resistant KB carcinoma cells. *Proceedings of the National Academy of Sciences of the Unites States of America*, *83*, 4538–4542.

Santarpia, M., González-Cao, M., Viteri, S., Karachaliou, N., Altavilla, G., & Rosell, R. (2015). Programmed cell death protein-1/programmed cell death ligand-1 pathway inhibition and predictive biomarkers: Understanding transforming growth factor-beta role. *Translational Lung Cancer Research*, *4*, 728–742.

Sarkar, D., Boukerche, H., Su, Z. Z., & Fisher, P. B. (2008). MDA-9/Syntenin: More than just a simple adapter protein when it comes to cancer metastasis. *Cancer Research*, *68*, 3087–3093.

Scatena, R., Bottoni, P., & Giardina, B. (2013). Circulating tumour cells and cancer stem cells: A role for proteomics in defining the interrelationships between function, phenotype and differentiation with potential clinical applications. *Biochimica et Biophysica Acta, 1835*, 129–143.

Schatton, T., & Frank, M. H. (2009). Antitumor immunity and cancer stem cells. *Annals of the New York Academy of Sciences, 1176*, 154–169.

Schempp, C. M., von Schwarzenberg, K., Schreiner, L., Kubisch, R., Müller, R., Wagner, E., et al. (2014). V-ATPase inhibition regulates anoikis resistance and metastasis of cancer cells. *Molecular Cancer Therapeutics, 13*, 926–937.

Schmidt, C. (2012). Cancer stem cells in the crosshairs. *Cancer Discovery, 2*, 384.

Schwitalla, S., Fingerle, A. A., Cammareri, P., Nebelsiek, T., Göktuna, S. I., Ziegler, P. K., et al. (2013). Intestinal tumorigenesis initiated by dedifferentiation and acquisition of stem-cell-like properties. *Cell, 152*, 25–38.

Sell, S. (2004). Stem cell origin of cancer and differentiation therapy. *Critical Reviews in Oncology/Hematology, 51*, 1–28.

Sell, S. (2010). On the stem cell origin of cancer. *The American Journal of Pathology, 176*, 2584–2594.

Shimono, Y., Zabala, M., Cho, R. W., Lobo, N., Dalerba, P., Qian, D., et al. (2009). Down-regulation of miRNA-200c links breast cancer stem cells with normal stem cells. *Cell, 138*, 592–603.

Shukla, S., & Meeran, S. M. (2014). Epigenetics of cancer stem cells: Pathways and therapeutics. *Biochimica et Biophysica Acta, 1840*, 3494–3502.

Simple, M., Suresh, A., Das, D., & Kuriakose, M. A. (2015). Cancer stem cells and field cancerization of oral squamous cell carcinoma. *Oral Oncology, 51*, 643–651.

Simpson, C. D., Anyiwe, K., & Schimmer, A. D. (2008). Anoikis resistance and tumor metastasis. *Cancer Letters, 272*, 177–185.

Song, S. J., Poliseno, L., Song, M. S., Ala, U., Webster, K., Ng, C., et al. (2013). MicroRNA-antagonism regulates breast cancer stemness and metastasis via TET-family-dependent chromatin remodeling. *Cell, 154*, 311–324.

Squadrito, M. L., & De Palma, M. (2015). A niche role for periostin and macrophages in glioblastoma. *Nature Cell Biology, 17*, 107–109.

Staudt, M. R., Sarkar, D., & Fisher, P. B. (2007). Differentiation therapy of cancer: Journey from the laboratory into the clinic. *Advances in Gene Molecular and Cell Therapy, 1*, 10–19.

Takebe, N., Miele, L., Harris, P. J., Jeong, W., Bando, H., Kahn, M., et al. (2015). Targeting Notch, Hedgehog, and Wnt pathways in cancer stem cells: Clinical update. *Nature Reviews. Clinical Oncology, 12*, 445–464.

Tang, D. G. (2012). Understanding cancer stem cell heterogeneity and plasticity. *Cell Research, 22*, 457–472.

Tarasova, N. I., Seth, R., Tarasov, S. G., Kosakowska-Cholody, T., Hrycyna, C. A., Gottesman, M. M., et al. (2005). Transmembrane inhibitors of P-glycoprotein, an ABC transporter. *Journal of Medicinal Chemistry, 48*, 3768–3775.

Toloudi, M., Apostolou, P., Chatziioannou, M., & Papasotiriou, I. (2011). Correlation between cancer stem cells and circulating tumor cells and their value. *Case Reports in Oncology, 4*, 44–54.

Tu, L. C., Foltz, G., Lin, E., Hood, L., & Tian, Q. (2009). Targeting stem cells-clinical implications for cancer therapy. *Current Stem Cell Research & Therapy, 4*, 147–153.

Vanharanta, S., & Massagué, J. (2012). Field cancerization: Something new under the sun. *Cell, 149*, 1179–1181.

Visvader, J. E., & Lindeman, G. J. (2012). Cancer stem cells: Current status and evolving complexities. *Cell Stem Cell, 10*, 717–728.

Wang, Q., Chen, Z. G., Du, C. Z., Wang, H. W., Yan, L., & Gu, J. (2009). Cancer stem cell marker CD133 + tumour cells and clinical outcome in rectal cancer. *Histopathology, 55*, 284–293.

Wang, X.-Y., & Fisher, P. B. (Eds.), (2015). Immunotherapy of cancer. Preface. *Advances in Cancer Research, 128,* xiii–xv. doi: 10.1016/S0065-230X(15)00086-X.

Wang, X.-Y., Zuo, D., Sarkar, D., & Fisher, P. B. (2011). Blockade of cytotoxic T-lymphocyte antigen-4 (CTLA-4) as a novel therapeutic approach for advanced melanoma. *Expert Opinion on Pharmacotherapy, 12,* 2695–2706.

Wongtrakoongate, P. (2015). Epigenetic therapy of cancer stem and progenitor cells by targeting DNA methylation machineries. *World Journal of Stem Cells, 7,* 137–148.

Yang, X., Lin, X., Zhong, X., Kaur, S., Li, N., Liang, S., et al. (2010). Double-negative feedback loop between reprogramming factor lin28 and microRNA let-7 regulates aldehyde dehydrogenase 1-positive cancer stem cells. *Cancer Research, 70,* 9463–9472.

Zhang, L., Tong, X., Li, J., Huang, Y., Hu, X., Chen, Y., et al. (2015). Apoptotic and autophagic pathways with relevant small-molecule compounds, in cancer stem cells. *Cell Proliferation, 48,* 385–397.

Zou, W. (2005). Immunosuppressive networks in the tumour environment and their therapeutic relevance. *Nature Reviews. Cancer, 5,* 263–274.

INDEX

Note: Page numbers followed by "*f*" indicate figures, and "*t*" indicate tables.

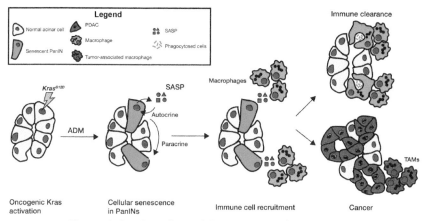

Fig. 1, A. Porciuncula *et al.* (See Page 11 of this volume.)

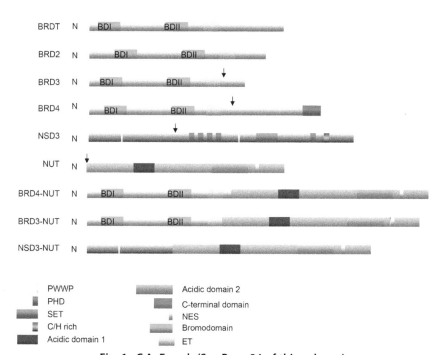

Fig. 1, C.A. French (See Page 24 of this volume.)

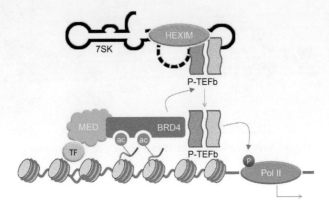

Fig. 2, C.A. French (See Page 25 of this volume.)

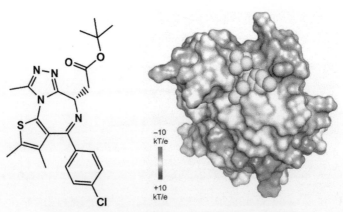

Fig. 3, C.A. French (See Page 33 of this volume.)

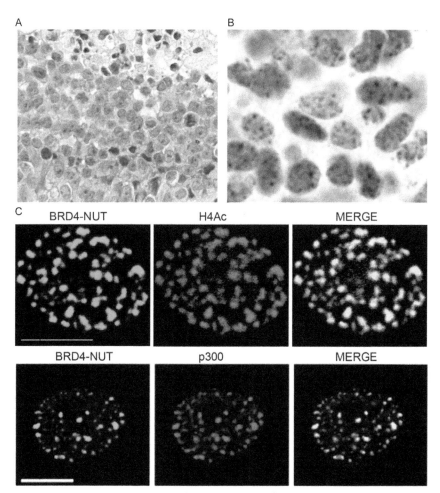

Fig. 4, C.A. French (See Page 37 of this volume.)

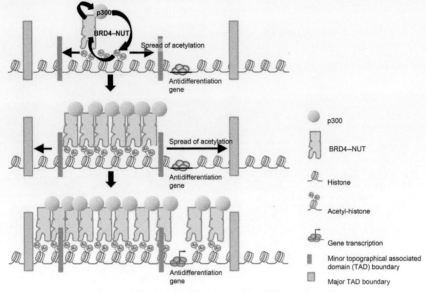

Fig. 5, C.A. French (See Page 42 of this volume.)

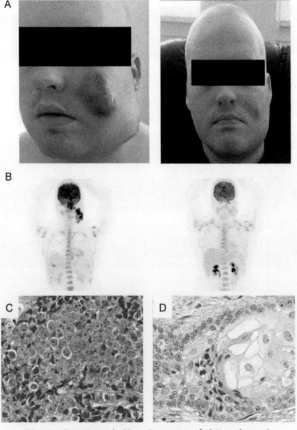

Fig. 6, C.A. French (See Page 44 of this volume.)

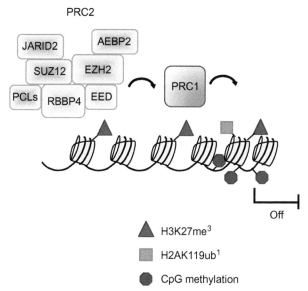

PRC2

H3K27me^3

H2AK119ub^1

CpG methylation

Fig. 1, J.N. Nichol et al. (See Page 61 of this volume.)

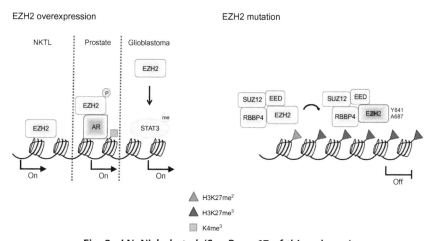

EZH2 overexpression

EZH2 mutation

NKTL   Prostate   Glioblastoma

H3K27me^2

H3K27me^3

K4me^3

Fig. 2, J.N. Nichol et al. (See Page 67 of this volume.)

H3K27me^3 reader mutations

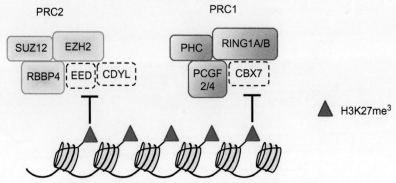

Fig. 3, J.N. Nichol *et al.* (See Page 70 of this volume.)

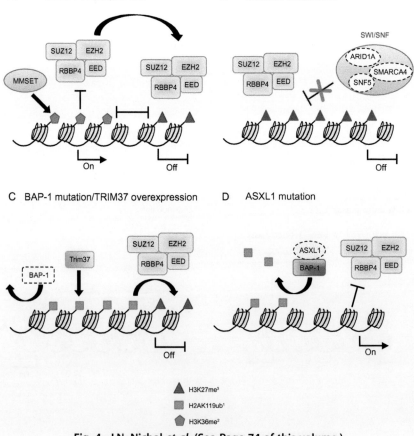

A MMSET overexpression

B SWI/SNF inactivation

C BAP-1 mutation/TRIM37 overexpression

D ASXL1 mutation

▲ H3K27me^3
■ H2AK119ub^1
⬠ H3K36me^2

Fig. 4, J.N. Nichol *et al.* (See Page 74 of this volume.)

Potential markers for response to inhibitors of H3K27 methylation

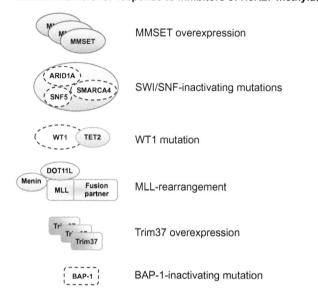

MMSET overexpression

SWI/SNF-inactivating mutations

WT1 mutation

MLL-rearrangement

Trim37 overexpression

BAP-1-inactivating mutation

Potential markers for response to inhibitors of H3K27 demethylation

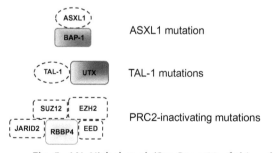

ASXL1 mutation

TAL-1 mutations

PRC2-inactivating mutations

Fig. 5, J.N. Nichol *et al.* (See Page 80 of this volume.)

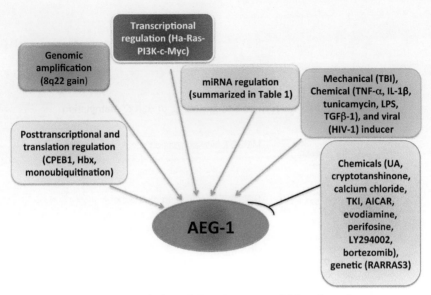

Fig. 1, L. Emdad *et al.* (See Page 100 of this volume.)

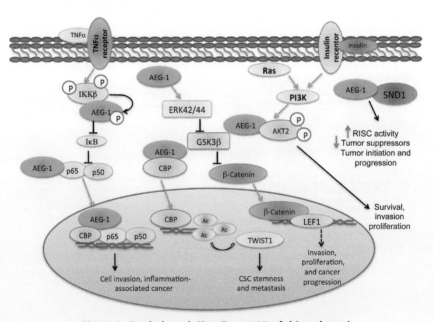

Fig. 2, L. Emdad *et al.* (See Page 107 of this volume.)

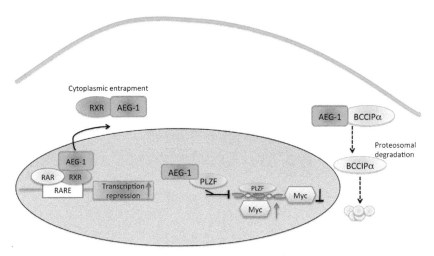

Fig. 3, L. Emdad *et al.* (See Page 113 of this volume.)

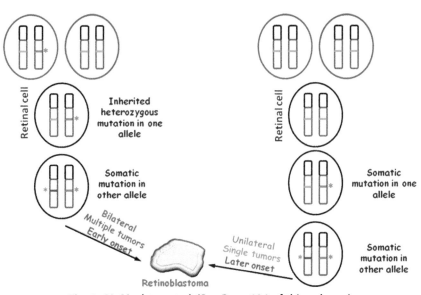

Fig. 1, M. Mushtaq *et al.* (See Page 134 of this volume.)

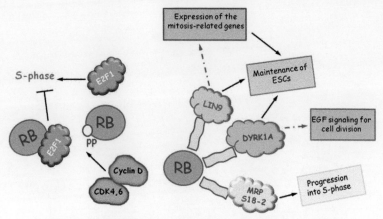

Fig. 2, M. Mushtaq *et al.* (See Page 136 of this volume.)

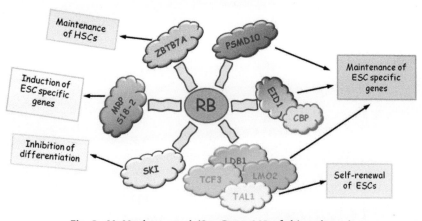

Fig. 3, M. Mushtaq *et al.* (See Page 143 of this volume.)

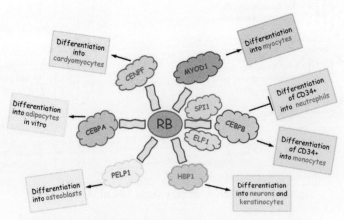

Fig. 4, M. Mushtaq *et al.* (See Page 147 of this volume.)

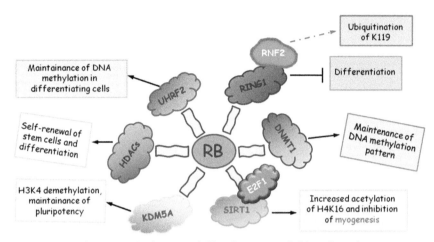

Fig. 5, M. Mushtaq *et al.* (See Page 150 of this volume.)

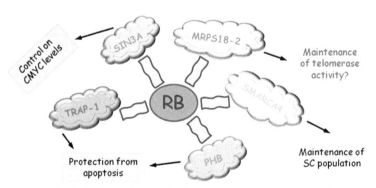

Fig. 6, M. Mushtaq *et al.* (See Page 152 of this volume.)

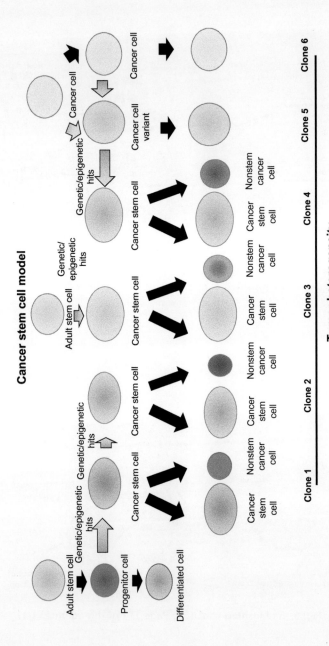

Fig. 1, S. Talukdar et al. (See Page 162 of this volume.)

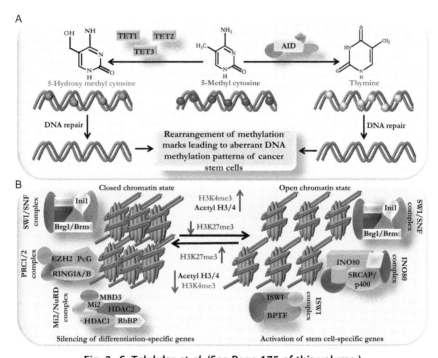

Fig. 2, S. Talukdar *et al.* (See Page 175 of this volume.)

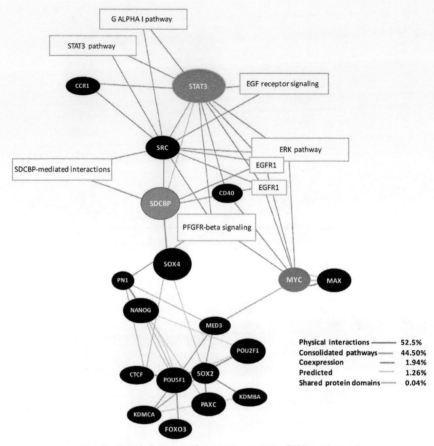

Fig. 3, S. Talukdar *et al.* (See Page 179 of this volume.)

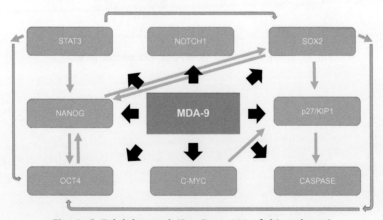

Fig. 4, S. Talukdar *et al.* (See Page 180 of this volume.)